Thwarting Consumer Choice

Thwarting Consumer Choice

The Case against Mandatory Labeling for Genetically Modified Foods

Gary E. Marchant, Guy A. Cardineau,
and Thomas P. Redick

The AEI Press

Publisher for the American Enterprise Institute

WASHINGTON, D.C.

Distributed by arrangement with the Rowman & Littlefield Publishing Group, 4501 Forbes Boulevard, Suite 200, Lanham, Maryland 20706. To order call toll free 1-800-462-6420 or 1-717-794-3800. For all other inquiries please contact AEI Press, 1150 Seventeenth Street, N.W. Washington, D.C. 20036 or call 1-800-862-5801.

NRI NATIONAL RESEARCH INITIATIVE

This publication is a project of the National Research Initiative, a program of the American Enterprise Institute that is designed to support, publish, and disseminate research by university-based scholars and other independent researchers who are engaged in the exploration of important public policy issues.

Library of Congress Cataloging-in-Publication Data

Marchant, Gary Elvin, 1958-
  Thwarting consumer choice : the case against mandatory labeling for genetically modified foods / Gary E. Marchant, Guy A. Cardineau, and Thomas P. Redick.
    p. cm.
  Includes bibliographical references and index.
  ISBN-13: 978-0-8447-4326-4
  ISBN-10: 0-8447-4326-7
  1. Genetically modified foods—Labeling. 2. Genetically modified foods—Law and legislation. I. Cardineau, Guy A. II. Redick, Thomas P. (Thomas Parker), 1959- III. Title.
  TP374.5.M36 2010
  363.19'29—dc22

                                                                2010003407

14 13 12 11 10   1 2 3 4 5 6 7

Printed in the United States of America

Contents

Acknowledgments

The authors appreciate the assistance of Marlin Walker and Kimball Nill.

PART I

Introduction and Background

Introduction

There is always an easy solution to every human problem—neat, plausible, and wrong.

—H. L. Mencken (1880–1956)

Demands for the mandatory labeling of genetically modified (GM) foods have become a central rallying cry of anti-GM activists in the United States and around the world. International, national, and local activist groups, such as Greenpeace, Friends of the Earth, and the Institute for Responsible Technology, have ongoing campaigns to impose mandatory GM labeling. The European Union (EU), having lost its World Trade Organization battle against the United States to block GM foods outright, is now enforcing a stringent traceability and labeling program for them that is the centerpiece of its prohibitive biotechnology regulatory regime.

Outside the EU, GM labeling requirements have been enacted in Australia, New Zealand, Japan, Korea, India, China, and several other nations in Africa, Asia, and Latin America. While these labeling laws are frequently unenforced and have no scientific justification, they have succeeded in stigmatizing and limiting the availability and benefits of GM foods. Anti-GM activists are actively campaigning to extend these restrictive labeling laws worldwide, including in the United States, and in 2009 launched a petition drive to pressure President Barack Obama to act on his purported "campaign promise" to require the mandatory labeling of GM foods.[1] (The allegation of such a promise by then-candidate Obama was later exposed as unfounded.)[2]

At first glance, several arguments in favor of mandatory labeling of GM foods are superficially compelling. People in a free society clearly should

3

have the choice of what types of products they purchase and consume. Markets generally work best when participants have more information rather than less, and labels on food are one way to deliver that information. From a democratic governance perspective, some public opinion polls claim that 90 percent or more of Americans support mandatory labeling of GM foods (at least when the costs of such a program are not mentioned). Why shouldn't the public's ostensible view prevail? Why should companies that trumpet the many benefits of biotechnology be afraid of a requirement to tell consumers which products contain these heralded products? As *Business Week* commented, "By blocking grassroots attempts to put advisory labels on food, the food and biotech industries look as if they have something to hide."[3] Finally, from an ethical perspective, shouldn't people have the right to know what is in their food?

In opposition to these superficially appealing contentions, this book digs deeper into the legal, ethical, and scientific arguments for mandatory GM labeling and finds that the reality is much different from the images presented by its proponents. We show that, contrary to the rhetoric of promoting consumer choice, GM labeling is actually being advocated as part of a strategy to block the availability of GM products as an option consumers may choose. Moreover, while often portrayed as a simple, essentially cost-free measure to add a few words to food labels, mandatory GM labeling in fact imposes substantial economic and liability costs and burdens along the entire food supply chain by requiring the segregation of GM from non-GM products at every stage from farm to fork. When consumers are asked a more balanced question that includes some recognition of the significant added costs of mandatory GM labeling, public opinion swings dramatically against it.

Moreover, the availability of clearly marked non-GM and organic foods through voluntary market forces provides consumers who prefer not to consume GM foods with the option to avoid them, without externalizing those costs onto other consumers, including the many lower-income citizens who would be disproportionately affected by the costs of mandatory GM labeling in industrialized countries. Even more tragic would be the impacts of mandatory GM labeling in denying populations in developing countries the many urgently needed benefits of food biotechnology.[4] Finally, from a fairness perspective, GM labeling would, without scientific justification, arbitrarily single out and stigmatize a relatively safe technology for disparate and unfair treatment. In short, the very arguments used to argue for mandatory GM food labeling—consumer choice, public opinion, and fairness— actually weigh against it when examined more closely.

The GM labeling saga provides a broader lesson about the dangers of an increasingly common demand by public interest groups to impose mandatory product labels based not on risk or science, but rather on sociopolitical goals and strategic agendas. Similar activist campaigns are already well underway or are emerging to mandate the stigmatizing and counterproductive labeling of, for example, irradiated foods, nanotechnology products, and foods derived from cloned animals (see appendix A on "Animal Cloning: The Latest Skirmish"). All of these campaigns have the potential to deter investment and innovation in promising emerging technologies and to deprive the public of beneficial new products. Consequently, the outcome of the GM food labeling controversy is likely to have repercussions and set precedents that will spread far beyond the field of biotechnology.

This book proceeds in three parts. Part I provides background on GM foods, including what is known about their benefits and risks, and then summarizes and compares current laws around the world mandating GM labels. Part II critically assesses the most common arguments advanced in support of mandatory GM labeling, and shows that each falls short in justifying—and in most cases actually weighs against—such labeling requirements. Finally, part III provides additional arguments against mandatory GM labeling, including the substantial costs, burdens, and disruptions associated with it, and the availability of a superior voluntary, market-based approach that will empower consumers to choose freely whether or not to purchase and consume GM foods.

1

Background on GM Foods

The controversy over the labeling of GM foods is primarily a surrogate bat-tleground for the larger issue of whether or not to permit the production of genetically modified foods. Before addressing the legal and policy issues relating to the labeling of GM foods, we provide this brief summary of GM technologies and foods developed by modern biotechnology, including their risks and benefits, as background for an evaluation of the stated rationales for mandatory labeling of GM foods.

Biotechnology Techniques

Modern biotechnology involves the use of molecular methods to add to, delete, or otherwise modify the DNA sequence of an organism. The development of recombinant DNA techniques in the 1970s enabled scientists to "cut and paste" DNA sequences at precise locations, and then to transfer selected DNA segments into the genomes of other organisms, including those from distantly related species. For some crops, a "gene gun" inserts the new genes using tiny "bullets" of DNA. The resulting "transgenic" or "genetically modified" (GM) organisms may express new or improved traits that can be beneficial for agricultural, nutritional, medical, or industrial applications.

The "genetic engineering" of GM crops and organisms made possible by modern biotechnology provides unprecedented power in terms of the speed and precision with which humans can genetically alter other species. At the same time, modern biotechnology is really only an extension (albeit far more efficient) of traditional methods of species modification that plant breeders have employed throughout human history. Going back many cen-turies, we find that farmers sought to improve their crops and farm animals through the process of selective breeding. These methods have been used to create many new types of crops that never existed naturally in nature, including modern corn, wheat, and canola.

In the twentieth century, the slow process of selective breeding was accelerated by the use of such techniques as chemical mutagenesis and irradiation, which have been used to generate improved crops with new genetic traits.[1] Over two thousand crop varieties commercialized to date have been created using chemical or radiation mutagenesis.[2] Some of these mutation-bred varieties have traits similar to existing GM crops, such as resistance to a particular herbicide. Mutation breeding produces genetic changes that are far less precise and certain than those possible with genetic engineering; as they are not targeted to specific genes, these methods simultaneously cause mutations in many other parts of the genome in addition to the gene of interest.[3] The National Academy of Sciences has noted that "a mutation made by traditional techniques may be accompanied by many unknown mutations, which often have deleterious effects on the organism."[4]

Traditional mutagenesis used to create many of our foods not only creates more genetic lesions than the more precise genetic engineering, but may create more risky genetic changes. Many mutagenesis-created genetic changes don't exist in nature and, accordingly, have never survived the screening of natural selection. In contrast, with genetic engineering, even the rare transference of a single gene from a distant species generally involves DNA that is genetically very similar to the host's own genes and has been demonstrated to be harmless by the rigors of millions of years of natural selection. The bottom line is that most foods we eat today have been "genetically modified" by humans, often using less precise methods than made possible by modern biotechnology. In fact, according to one account, only four crops grown in North America today were not originally adapted from other regions of the world—the blueberry, Jerusalem artichoke, sunflower, and squash.[5]

GM Crops and Foods

While biotechnology has been used to manufacture a wide range of pharmaceuticals, industrial products, and, most recently, transgenic animals, arguably its most successful commercial application to date has been the development of genetically modified crops used for food, fuel, fiber, and animal feed. At present, most efforts directed at the genetic engineering of crops relate to addressing so-called "input" traits—those that help the food producer to lower the cost of production and increase yield. Examples include adding traits that provide resistance to insects, tolerance to herbicides, resistance to disease (viral, bacterial, and fungal), and resistance to stress (salt, drought, heat, and cold). Insect resistance and herbicide tolerance were the first major commercial GM traits, entering the marketplace in 1996. GM crops have proved very popular with farmers because of their advantages, and, in 2008, over 300 million acres of land in twenty-five different countries were planted with them.[6] In the United States, approximately 91 percent of the soybeans, 88 percent of the cotton, and 85 percent of the corn grown in 2009 were GM varieties.[7]

This first generation of GM crops has not only reduced costs and increased yield, but has also produced demonstrated environmental benefits, including reduced pesticide use, shifts to less environmentally harmful herbicides, a reduction in the environmentally destructive tilling of soils, increased protection of water quality through reduced soil erosion and runoff, reduced greenhouse gas emissions (from less plowing and fewer herbicide applications), and less destruction of natural habitat (by increasing yield from existing cultivated lands).[8] For example, one recent study calculated that in the decade 1996–2005, GM crops reduced pesticide sprayings worldwide by 493 million pounds (a 7 percent overall reduction), decreased the adverse environmental impacts of pesticides by 15 percent, and reduced global warming emissions by an amount equivalent to the reduction that would be achieved by removing 4 million cars from the road for one year.[9]

"Output" traits involve improvements to the food product itself rather than the method of growing it and are projected to enhance consumer acceptance by offering benefits consumers can directly enjoy, such as healthier or tastier foods. The pipeline of new biotech crops is packed with varieties that have improved protein and oil profiles and fiber composition, and increased vitamin content. One of the most compelling new crops exhibiting output traits is the so-called "Golden Rice," which has the potential to help address Vitamin A deficiency in millions of people in developing nations who consume rice as their principal staple food. Vitamin A deficiency leads to blindness and exacerbates other conditions, such as respiratory diseases and diarrhea.[10]

Other output traits under development will lead to the engineering of plants to produce drugs and other value-added medical products. Plant-based vaccines that can be delivered orally have the potential both to be inexpensively produced and to eliminate the need for refrigeration and sterile needles.[11] Another significant area of research and development, the improvement of biofuel production, applies genetic engineering to obtaining biodiesel from plant oils and bioethanol from corn and sugar-cane,[12] with biotech enzymes perhaps enhancing the conversion of cellulose to ethanol and bringing long-awaited "cellulosic" ethanol into broad commercial production.

In summary, biotechnology is offering a growing number of consumer-centered products, as well as new agronomic traits that increase yield and reduce production costs and environmental harms. From a production standpoint, GM crops are an unqualified success, and they are now on the verge of becoming a consumer success as well.

Risks of GM Crops and Foods

There are few, if any, technologies whose risks have generated as much smoke and as little fire as the genetic modification of foods. Despite hundreds of published, peer-reviewed studies,[13] thousands of safety tests, numerous false alarms seized on by activist groups only to be found unwarranted, almost two billion acres of GM plants cultivated,[14] and an estimated one trillion GM meals eaten, not one case of harm to human health or the environment from GM crops or foods has been documented.[15] At a time of almost daily media reports about real food risks from contaminated spinach, unpasteurized milk, tainted peanut butter and pistachios, hazardous residues in imported foods, and food allergies, the pristine safety record of GM foods is a remarkable and underreported achievement. As National Academy of Sciences member Dr. Nina Federoff noted, GM crops may well be "the safest technology that human beings have ever invented."[16]

This safety record is all the more impressive given the intense and generally sensational media scrutiny of GM foods and the fact that companies developing GM products routinely spend millions of dollars on safety testing for each new product, including tests that look for changes in allergenicity, toxicity, and nutrient composition, as well as ecological risks and any unintended effects.[17] This evaluation ensures that new biotech plants bound for food use are just as safe as—or safer than—the same plants using traditional breeding methods. In contrast to this rigorous risk assessment of GM crops, relatively few analytical studies are done on new conventional (or organic) varieties of crops—even ones that are created using mutagenesis methods to induce traits similar to those found in many GM crops, such as herbicide resistance.

Every major scientific organization that has examined the issue has concluded that GM crops and foods as a category present no greater risks than their conventional counterparts. For example, the U.S. Food and Drug Administration (FDA) found no evidence that GM foods as a category are any riskier than conventional foods.[18] Similarly, the U.S. National Academy of Sciences concluded in 2000 that "there is no strict dichotomy between, or new categories of, the health and environmental risks that might be posed by transgenic and conventional . . . plants,"[19] and reaffirmed in 2002 that "the transgenic process presents no new categories of risk compared to conventional methods of crop improvement."[20]

At the international level, a joint expert consultation by the World Health Organization (WHO) and the Food and Agriculture Organization (FAO) concluded in 1996 that changes made by genetic engineering are "basically of the same nature as those that might arise from other ways of altering the genome of an organism, such as conventional breeding."[21] WHO elsewhere states:

> GM foods currently available on the international market have passed risk assessments and are not likely to present risks for human health. In addition, no effects on human health have been shown as a result of the consumption of such foods by the general population in the countries where they have been approved.[22]

In yet another report, the FAO further endorses the safety of GM foods, noting that such foods have been assessed for increased risks to human health by several national regulatory authorities (*inter alia,* Argentina, Brazil, Canada, China, the United Kingdom, and the United States) using their national food safety procedures. To date, no verifiable untoward toxic or nutritionally deleterious effects resulting from the consumption of foods derived from genetically modified crops have been discovered anywhere in the world. Many millions of people have consumed foods derived from genetically modified plants . . . without any observed adverse effects.[23]

Even the European Union's own scientific advisors concluded in 2001 that the "use of more precise technology and the greater regulatory scrutiny probably make (GM foods and crops) even safer than conventional plants and foods."[24]

Given this history of safe use and the steady increase in plantings (approximately 10 percent annually), the tide of mandatory GM food labeling laws may be reaching its highwater mark. Nations that adopt such requirements merely to enhance prospects for trade with some markets may find the net benefit of such trade outweighed by the negative impacts to health, environment, and economy that arise from GM food labeling laws. As this book will argue, nations that have adopted mandatory GM labeling laws should reassess their choices in light of newly emerging evidence on the proven benefits, strong safety record, and growing acceptability of GM crops. The next chapter reviews the various labeling laws now on the books around the world, describes the troublesome differences among such laws, and analyzes their status under the broader scheme of international trade law.

2

GM Labeling Laws and Regulations

For almost two decades, controversy has raged in almost every corner of the planet on whether labeling should be made mandatory for GM foods. The United States is the leading nation opposing mandatory labeling, while the European Union is its leading proponent. Numerous other countries have adopted or are debating the adoption of labeling requirements, and, as of the date of this writing, at least forty-six nations (see appendix B) had imposed them (although the requirements are often enforced poorly or not at all outside the EU, Japan, Australia, and other developed nations).

This chapter first summarizes the history and status of the GM labeling debate and any resulting labeling laws in the United States, EU, and other nations in Asia, Africa, and Latin America. It then provides a brief analysis of key design features and differences in the requirements of different countries that have adopted mandatory GM labeling. Finally, it briefly explores the status and legality of GM labeling requirements under international trade law.

Status and History of Mandatory GM Labeling Requirements

The legal foundation of mandatory "GM" labeling of food begins with a "precautionary approach" to the safety of biotech crops—a legal principle that the European Union applies to a logical extreme, while the United States rejects it. There is a stark contrast between the voluntary labeling approach taken in the United States—which provides the optimum level of choice for all consumers—and the EU approach, which uses mandatory GM food labeling to serve "collective preferences" and the consumer's "right to know" about processes used in creating their food. In pursuit of this precautionary approach, the EU is raising the costs of food, including meat products, for its consuming public, with no discernible health or environmental benefits for those consumers.

United States. In 1986, as the first GM products were beginning to move out of the laboratory and into the field-testing stage, the United States government issued the "coordinated framework" for the regulation of biotechnology that remains in effect today.[1] The coordinated framework distributes regulatory responsibility for the safety of biotechnology products among several federal agencies, depending on the nature of the product and the type of activity being pursued (that is, research, field testing, commercial horticulture, food processing, or marketing). The U.S. Food and Drug Administration (FDA) is assigned responsibility for ensuring the safety of foods produced using biotechnology under its authority provided by the Federal Food, Drug and Cosmetic Act (FFDCA), and therefore is also responsible for deciding whether GM foods should be labeled.

In 1992, the FDA issued a policy document laying out its approach for regulating GM foods, which remains largely unchanged today.[2] The agency adopted the principle of "substantial equivalence" to govern its approach to GM foods, which has been defined by the Organisation of Economic Cooperation and Development (OECD) as follows:

> The concept of substantial equivalence embodies the idea that existing organisms used as foods, or as a source of food, can be used as the basis for comparison when assessing the safety of human consumption of a food or food component that has been modified or is new.[3]

Under this "substantial equivalence" approach, GM foods that are sufficiently similar to existing foods would not be subject to greater regulatory scrutiny.

The FDA determined that, consistent with longstanding agency labeling precedent and policy as well as the principle of substantial equivalence, labeling would only be required and appropriate for "material" facts about a food product.[4] The FDA has been very careful over the decades to avoid cluttering food labels with nonessential information:

For more than 60 years, the FDA has had in its enforcement and policymaking arsenal [the] authority to require information to appear on the food label. The agency has exercised that authority sparingly, largely reserving its use for the disclosure of truly important, noncollateral and non-label-cluttering "material" information. The food label would be an entirely different entity from what it is today if the FDA had acted otherwise. For example, imagine the possible array of different types of information that could be "required" if the FDA deemed "public desire" for information as an indicator of materiality. And, further, imagine the possibly unworkable contours, not to mention the size and space demands, of a label capable of accommodating such information.[5]

Applying this longstanding and legally validated approach to GM foods, which, the FDA concluded, presented no greater risks than any other type of food, the agency rejected calls for mandatory labeling, finding that the fact that a food was made using genetic engineering was not "material" information:

The agency is not aware of any information showing that foods derived by these new methods differ from other foods in any meaningful or uniform way, or that, as a class, foods developed by the new techniques present any different or greater safety concern than foods developed by traditional plant breeding. For this reason, the agency does not believe that the method of development of a new plant variety (including the use of new techniques including recombinant DNA techniques) is normally material information within the meaning of [the FFDCA] and would not usually be required to be disclosed in labeling for the food.[6]

The FDA's policy on food labeling would, however, require labeling if a genetically modified food were found by scientific evidence to present "material" novel risks, such as allergenicity or toxicity. The FDA stated that "consumers must be informed, by appropriate labeling, if a food derived from [genetic engineering] differs from its traditional counterpart such that the common or usual name no longer applies to the food, or if a safety or usage issue exists to which consumers must be alerted."[7]

The FDA's decision not to require GM food labeling was challenged in federal district court by a coalition of citizen groups who attacked the FDA position on a variety of grounds, all of which were rejected by the court. The district court upheld the FDA's determination that the mere fact that GM foods were produced using genetic engineering was not "material" information whose inclusion on the label was required under the FFDCA or long-standing precedent.[8] The court also rejected the challengers' claim that the FDA was required to consider "widespread consumer interest" in favor of labeling as a relevant factor:

> Plaintiffs fail to understand the limitation on the FDA's power to consider consumer demand when making labeling decisions because they fail to recognize that the determination that a product differs materially from the type of product it purports to be is a factual predicate to the requirement of labeling. Only once materiality has been established may the FDA consider consumer opinion to determine whether a label is required to disclose a material fact. Thus "if there is a [material] difference, and consumers would like to know about the difference, then labeling is appropriate. If, however, the product does not differ in any significant way from what it purports to be, then it would be misbranding to label the product as different, even if consumers misperceived the product as different."[9]

Since its 1992 decision rejecting mandatory labeling of GM foods, the FDA has been continuously pressured by various actors to change its policy, but it has held fast to its position under both Republican and Democratic administrations. Activist groups such as the Institute for Responsible Technology and the International Organic Consumers Association, often supported by organic food interests, have conducted a grassroots advocacy campaign in favor of mandatory GM labeling in the United States for many years without success.[10] Congressman Dennis Kucinich (D-Ohio) has introduced legislation entitled the "Genetically Engineered Food Right to Know Act" in each Congress since 1999 to require labeling of genetically engineered foods (the most recent bill had seventeen cosponsors), but to date no federal legislation has advanced.[11]

Attempts to impose mandatory GM labeling at the state level have also failed to pass. In 2002, Oregonians voted down a statewide proposition to mandate GM labeling. Even though public opinion was initially heavily in favor of the proposition, Oregon voters opted by a wide margin to continue to use voluntary non-GM labeling.[12] Vermont and Maine have also attempted to mandate GM labeling by state legislation. Any such requirement would likely face a preemption challenge as a result of the FDA's rejection of mandatory GM labeling.

Activist groups incorrectly claimed to have obtained commitments from *every* Democratic contender for the 2008 presidential primary nomination to support mandatory GM labeling[13] and, as noted above, launched a petition campaign pressuring President Obama to follow through on a promise he never made to require it.

European Union (EU). The EU has imposed the world's most stringent GM labeling requirements. In 1997, the EU first enacted its 1997 "Novel Food Law," which required the labeling of any food products with detectable GM residues exceeding a concentration ("tolerance") of 1.0 percent of the final product.[14] This original labeling program did not require labeling of products manufactured from GM ingredients which did not contain detectable amounts of modified DNA or proteins, such as many oils and other highly processed foods. In 2003, the EU adopted a more stringent traceability and labeling regime for biotech crops, which went into effect on April 18, 2004, and required labeling of any food products made from GM ingredients above a threshold of 0.9 percent, even if the modified ingredients could not be detected in the final product.[15] The 0.9 percent threshold only applied to the "adventitious presence" of EU-approved GM ingredients, and thus would only apply if the seller made a good-faith effort to keep out GM content. Otherwise, any level of unauthorized GM content or deliberate addition of an approved GM ingredient would trigger labeling (and potentially other) requirements. This "zero tolerance" policy toward GM products not authorized in the EU but approved in other nations imposed, as will be discussed later in chapter 7, extremely onerous burdens on exporting nations and companies.

The EU labeling law thus extended the scope of GM labeling requirements to all products derived "from" GM organisms, irrespective of the
detectability of DNA or protein in the final product. Various food products
contain ingredients "from" GM crops, including the "oilseeds" (soybean,
canola, and cottonseed oils), corn products (starch, glucose, high fructose
corn syrup, and ascorbic acid), soy lecithin, sterol, and other derived products. These processed, GM-free products made "from" GM plants are func-
tionally and physically identical to conventional versions of the same
products, but are now required to be labeled in the EU. To be able to enforce
this labeling requirement for foods that had no detectable GM content, the
2004 regulations also imposed a "farm to fork" traceability requirement that
mandated keeping a record of each GM ingredient at every step of the food
production process. Any entity in the food chain of a GM product is
required to maintain records for five years and is subject to audit to ensure
compliance. This document retention requirement operates to transfer
liability back along the food chain if a non-GM shipment fails to meet the
0.9 percent tolerance for adventitious presence (including presence of
detectable traces that "should have" been detected), or contains unap-
proved-in-EU genetic modifications.[16]

The EU's regulation adopting this labeling and traceability regime
expressly states that its purpose is "to ensure that consumers are fully and
reliably informed about GMOs [genetically modified organisms] and the
products, foods and feed produced therefrom, so as to allow them to make
an informed choice of product."[17] Yet, despite this avowed objective, the
regulations notably exempt foods made "with" contained uses of GM
microbes, such as cheeses made "with" genetically engineered chymosin
or beers made "with" GM yeast. The only apparent scientific distinction is
that these products are produced by large EU manufacturers (such as
Novo Nordisk), and they are commercially important to many EU
national economies.

This distinction exposes the protectionist hole in the logic of the EU's
mandatory GM food labeling regulations. Thus, when the EU requires labeling of products produced "from" GM organisms (such as soybean oil from
highly productive U.S. farms), but not labeling of products produced "with"
GM organisms (the beer and cheese so dear to EU hearts), its policy arguments about the consumer's "right to know" are revealed as disingenuous at

best. The EU regulations also do not require labeling of meat, milk, and other products from animals fed with GM feed—another instance, as with soybean oil, where the "process" does not leave any GM residue to trigger health concerns. In February 2007, Greenpeace delivered a petition with over one million European signatures calling on the EU regulators to expand the labeling requirement to milk, meat, eggs, and other animal products from animals that were fed with genetically modified organisms (GMOs),[18] and in October 2008 the Nordic Council called for tighter GM labeling in the Nordic region of Europe to include such applications.[19]

Other Nations. As listed in appendix B, at least forty-six nations (including all twenty-seven EU member states) have adopted mandatory GM labeling laws as of October 2009. Several other nations have pending GM labeling proposals, some of which have languished for years. These labeling requirements have been adopted by many important trading partners of the United States, including the EU, Japan, South Korea, Australia, Taiwan, and Russia. Other than in the EU nations, implementation and enforcement in many of the nations that mandate GM labeling is spotty at best, particularly in developing nations using GM crops that lack the resources required to test for low levels of GM content.[20]

While some developing nations, such as Brazil and Ecuador, have adopted mandatory GM labeling laws, there are signs that the tide may be turning against GM food labeling in the developing world. Nations across the Southern Hemisphere are reassessing the high cost of adopting a mandatory GM food labeling system.[21] Of those developing nations that have passed mandatory GM food labeling laws, nearly all fall short in offering necessary regulatory guidance to implement them, at times failing to set a commercial tolerance.[22]

In some cases, this lack of enforcement reflects uncertainty regarding the need for mandatory GM food labeling and the costs it might impose. India, for example, issued a GM labeling regulation that was to take effect on March 31, 2006, but delayed implementation pending a thorough review of the costs and necessity for such an approach.[23] Similar pauses to reflect on the implementation or enforcement of GM labeling policies have been seen in the past few years in Chile, Saudi Arabia, Sri Lanka, South Africa, and China, exhibiting varying degrees of indecisiveness.[24]

Key Design Issues and Differences in National Labeling Laws

Important and frequent inconsistencies occur in the GM labeling laws that have been adopted by various jurisdictions, greatly complicating compliance by food distributors operating in a global marketplace.[25] One important difference pertains to the applicable threshold for trace amounts of unintended GM content that are exempt from labeling. Several nations (for example, Indonesia, Taiwan, Japan, and Thailand) apply a 5 percent tolerance for approved GM content in non-GMO imports. In contrast, the EU and some other jurisdictions apply a much stricter tolerance of 0.9 percent for unintentional contamination of approved GM products. Such low tolerances are commercially less feasible to achieve in practice in nations that grow and export some GM crops. To confuse matters further, other nations have tolerance levels that are yet again different, such as Malaysia, which has enacted a still-pending implementation tolerance of 3 percent. These thresholds are not based on any scientific evidence indicating that levels of GM content above the tolerance are any more dangerous than levels just below it, but simply reflect particular governments' arbitrary decisions, based entirely on feasibility of detection, costs of testing, and political factors, and not supported by any risk-assessment process.[26]

Another major difference among national labeling laws is the scope of the requirement. Only European nations and Brazil, China, and Ecuador have laws that require GM labels for processed foods like canola or soybean oil that were produced "from" biotech crops but do not contain any detectable DNA or protein. These jurisdictions require labeling where no GM residues can be detected in the food product, in contrast to the labeling laws of other countries such as Japan, Australia, New Zealand, and Korea. The broader EU-type approach is obviously much more difficult to enforce, since review of a documentary trail is the only viable means of ascertaining the use of GM ingredients that are not detectable in the final product.

There are other differences in national labeling laws in terms of coverage. Some Asian nations (Thailand, Japan, and China, for instance) only require labeling if the ingredients listed on the label or the top three or five listed ingredients are genetically modified, whereas other national laws apply to all ingredients in a food product. Korea's GM labeling law only applies to packaged food, while others apply to both packaged and unpackaged food. New

Zealand requires labeling of food made "with" genetically engineered microbes; the EU and many other countries currently do not. The EU requires labeling of genetically modified animal feed; other countries do not. Some national laws apply to foods served by restaurants and caterers; others do not.

At the boundary of laws imposing mandatory GM food labeling, we have meat products. Currently, no nation requires labeling of meat, milk, or eggs produced from animals fed genetically modified grains, although activists around the world are pushing for such a requirement. Like the labeling of oils produced from biotech crops, the labeling of animal products would extend GM labeling beyond concern over food safety into the realm of policies that promote environmental causes (like dolphin-safe tuna). As will be discussed in chapter 7, this checkerboard pattern of inconsistent national GM labeling laws imposes a dizzying array of varying requirements that create substantial uncertainties, burdens, disruptions, and legal risks for global food producers and distributors.

International Law Fora

The controversy over mandatory GM labeling is also playing out in several international fora and multilateral environmental agreements. The Cartagena Protocol to the Convention on Biological Diversity opened for signature in 2000 and entered into force with the fiftieth signature on September 11, 2003. International shipments of genetically modified seeds for planting purposes require "advance informed agreement" (submission of dossiers on environmental health and safety by the exporting entity, followed by consent to the shipment by the importing country). For food and feed, however, a more streamlined process requires only that shipments state they "may contain" biotech crops, subject to any national import laws that seek more detailed information. [27]

For imports of food and feed bound for processing, this law was expanded in 2006 to require potentially more detailed notice of international shipments of products containing GM ingredients under Biosafety Protocol Article 18.2(a).[28] Also included is an obligation to state on commercial invoices that shipping containers "may contain" genetically modified products. While this labeling requirement does not apply to the product itself, nations such as Malaysia are implementing the Biosafety Protocol with GM labeling,[29] using this initial disclosure to set up labeling that consumers would see in the stores.

An ongoing controversy raised by disclosure requirements under Article 18.2(a) involves whether a shipper can simply state on the container label that this container "may" contain GM content, or whether it is required to verify and characterize the specific GM content of the shipment. In 2006, an interim compromise was reached, under which products with GM content that is tracked through an "identity preservation system" (an existing system of documentation and storage-related requirements intended to ensure that a product retains particular characteristics) shall be labeled as "containing" GM, while labeling on all other shipments can continue to say they "may contain" unspecified biotech ingredients, at least until the issue is revisited in the 2010 "Fifth Meeting of the Parties" in Nagoya, Japan.[30]

A major complication with the Cartagena Protocol is that most of the major GM exporting nations, including the United States, Canada, Argentina, and Australia, are not parties to it, and thus are not subject to the container labeling requirements. Nevertheless, the protocol is currently used to support GM labeling, by requiring shipments to state generally where they "may contain" GM crops. Implementation of the Biosafety Protocol through "biosafety laws" that contain added GM labeling rules is likely to have a significant impact on GM labeling programs for consumers.

Another international forum in which GM labeling has been debated is the Codex Alimentarius Commission, which sets consensus-based voluntary standards for food safety and quality under the auspices of the Food and Agriculture Organization (FAO). While national compliance with them is voluntary, Codex standards are given deference by the World Trade Organization in resolving international trade disputes. Codex's Committee on Food Labelling has been attempting to develop a standard for labeling of GM foods for over a decade, but efforts to reach consensus have been frustrated by the major differences in the positions of countries opposed to mandatory labeling, such as the United States, and pro-labeling members, such as the EU.

The third international forum in which GM labeling issues may be debated, but where they have not yet been directly presented, is the World Trade Organization (WTO). WTO requirements prohibit signatory nations from unduly restricting or impeding international trade with barriers that are not scientifically justified or necessary. It is possible that restrictive GM labeling laws such as those of the EU, which tend to have a protectionist effect and are based on a "precautionary approach," could be challenged under the WTO dispute resolution provisions. So far, the only challenge to laws regulating GM products was a WTO decision in 2006 granting relief to the United States, Canada, and Argentina from the inordinate delays of the EU in approving various biotech crop food and feed import applications submitted to its regulatory approval process.[31]

While U.S.-based commodity groups continue to call for a similar challenge to the EU's GM food labeling law, no action has been taken to date. In 2000, the United States warned the EU that it was considering making another formal complaint to the WTO in Geneva on the grounds that labeling GM products unlawfully discriminated against biotech crops, giving rise to an illegal restraint of trade.[32] While such a legal challenge has not been brought by the United States to date, such a claim would have a reasonable likelihood of success given the lack of any legitimate safety basis for a mandatory GM label, but it would raise some complex issues of first impression in world trade jurisprudence.

Under WTO law, nations can pass labeling laws that are "necessary" to protect human, animal, or plant life and health, provided they base such rules on scientific evidence. WTO rules generally require food labels intended to warn of health risks to take an approach based on scientifically verifiable risks associated with the content of the product, rather than an arbitrary focus on the process used in producing it.[33] Given that no national government that has adopted mandatory GM labeling to date has demonstrated or even tried to argue that GM products are inherently more risky than non-GM products, but rather have defended their requirements based on consumer choice and right-to-know arguments, mandatory GM labeling laws may run afoul of the WTO obligations. *EC Hormones Concerning Meat and Meat Products* (the "beef hormone case"), in which the United States successfully challenged the EU's prohibition of imports of U.S. hormone-fed beef, established that a country cannot base trade restrictions on the "precautionary principle" and on consumer preferences without showing some objective scientific evidence of food safety risks.[34] The latest decision in the string of decisions in the beef hormone case has reportedly recognized some role for "minority" scientific opinion, which some scholars see as an opening for increased allowance of precautionary *provisional* measures (temporary moves in the face of uncertainty), despite the fact that "the WTO has officially declared, in several of its Panel and Appellate Body Reports, that the precautionary principle has not been written into the SPS Agreement."[35]

Moreover, a nation enacting a requirement that restricts international trade must demonstrate that it is adopting the "least restrictive" measure. The availability of a less burdensome and minimally trade-restrictive, voluntary non-GM labeling measure (see chapter 8) to serve the stated objective of ensuring consumer choice would further undermine the EU's defense of its mandatory GM labeling scheme. Under this alternative, food suppliers and retailers could market products without GM content with a voluntary "Non-GM" label to provide the consumer choice the EU claims its GM labeling requirement is intended to fulfill. Voluntary labels would generally be considered less trade-restrictive than mandatory national laws.[36]

An additional tactic the United States could use to challenge the EU would be to attack the deliberately discriminatory and protectionist design of the EU's mandatory GM labeling regime. The labeling of one process— foods "from" GM crops—while excluding foods made "with" GM microbes is both scientifically indefensible and blatantly protectionist toward local interests (that is, the EU-based enzyme and food additive industry, which has products made "with" GM-microbes that are inherently no less risky than products made "from" GM crops that are required to be labeled). It follows that the decision to exclude the GMO microbes appears purely protectionist—discriminating against importers with a burdensome labeling and traceability regime while carefully exempting certain products to leave major EU industries untouched.[37]

In sum, the EU's mandatory GM labeling and traceability requirement likely violates world trade laws as a protectionist measure that restricts global trade because it imposes undue burdens on its trading partners and is unsupported by any objective scientific evidence of risk. Moreover, it is justified by an impermissible rationale standing apart from alleged consumer choice that could be addressed with a less burdensome voluntary alternative, and is selectively applied to some foods produced using GM technologies but not others without any rational justification other than protectionism and economic self-interest.

PART II

Critique of the Arguments for Mandatory GM Labeling

3

The "Right to Know"

A legitimate use of mandatory food labeling would be to warn consumers about real food risks. For example, foods containing peanuts are labeled to warn citizens with peanut allergies, and diet sodas are labeled with a warning that they contain phenylalanine, which can be dangerous to people with the genetic condition phenylketonuria (PKU). Thus, a conceivable argument for mandatory labeling of GM foods would be to warn consumers about potential health risks from such foods.[1] Indeed, some ethicists argue that this is the only circumstance in which a manufacturer has a responsibility to label its product.[2]

This potential "warning" rationale has no relevance for GM food labeling, however, because, as discussed in chapter 1, scientific expert bodies around the world have consistently reached the conclusion that GM foods as a category present no greater or unique risks relative to any other type of foods. In its 1992 GM policy statement, the FDA stated that, as with conventional foods, a warning label would be required if a GM food contained elevated levels of a potential allergen or toxin, or had changes in the levels of major dietary nutrients relative to unmodified forms of the same food.[3] No such labels have been required to date. Moreover, as many experts in both government and industry have reaffirmed, if a GM food does present significant human health risks, those risks should be regulated and controlled directly, rather than by simply warning consumers in a cryptic label about the particular process used in its creation.[4]

Accordingly, there is no health risk rationale for mandating the labeling of all GM foods, and no national government has relied on such a rationale to enact a mandatory GM labeling regime to date. The EU, for example, expressly disavowed any health warning purpose for its mandatory labeling regime promulgated in 2004. In the words of one EU official: "Safety is not the issue here."[5]

What, then, is the intended purpose of mandatory GM food labeling? Governments, activist organizations, and some scholars have offered a variety of purported rationales for mandatory GM labeling, often mixing and blurring these rationales together in a hodgepodge of argumentation. The most commonly advanced justifications for mandatory GM labeling are the overlapping themes of respecting the consumer's "right to know," providing "consumer choice," and adhering to public opinion. When examined individually, however, none of these rationales stands up to critical scrutiny. These and the other arguments advanced to support mandatory GM labeling are critically evaluated in the next four chapters, beginning with the "right to know" argument presented in this chapter.

The consumer's purported "right to know" is the most frequently invoked, and perhaps the most appealing, argument for mandatory GM labeling.[6] As a top EU regulator stated when the EU adopted its current GM labeling and traceability requirements, "Labeling serves the purpose of informing consumers and users and allowing them to exercise choice."[7] Similarly, on the other side of the Atlantic, the mandatory GM labeling legislation introduced in the U.S. Congress in 2006 by Representative Kucinich was titled "The Genetic Engineering Right to Know Act," and asserted that "consumers have a right to know whether the food they purchase contains or was produced with genetically engineered material."[8]

Giving individuals information so that they can make informed choices based on their own preferences is a fundamental tenet of free markets. Accordingly, informing consumers as to which food products contain genetic modifications would seem to be consistent with both market principles and individual autonomy, empowering consumers to act with their pocketbooks in choosing whether or not to buy GM foods.[9] While this argument may seem compelling at a superficial level, deeper scrutiny demonstrates that mandatory GM labeling fails to fulfill any meaningful right to know.

To begin with, all GM foods carry the same generic label (for example, "Contains genetically modified organisms") under all existing mandatory labeling programs. In an attempt to get around prohibitive costs, some proponents of mandatory GM labeling based on consumer autonomy principles propose an even weaker labeling scheme in which GM foods need not be segregated, tracked, and tested; rather, any food item not known for certain to be non-GM must carry a generic "may contain" GM label.[10]

These weak labeling schemes—the only ones that seem to be economically viable—fail to satisfy any meaningful consumer autonomy demands. The Nuffeld Council on Bioethics, in its comprehensive review of the ethical issues associated with GM foods, concluded that "labeling is meaningless unless the public knows what genetic modification is."[11] Moreover, with such general statements, consumers would not have the choice of avoiding only those specific GM foods to which they object; their only option would be to avoid all GM-labeled food.[12] Public opinion surveys show that the public wants additional information in order to differentiate GM food products by their properties and benefits, and that a label stating simply that the product contains GM ingredients would be of limited usefulness to most consumers.[13]

Even the limited option of simply knowing whether or not a food product contains GM ingredients would not truly be available. All mandatory GM labeling schemes enacted to date have a threshold or tolerance of GM content that triggers the labeling requirement, and, in fact, any requirement without such a tolerance would be infeasible. Consequently, many foods without a GM label may, indeed, contain GM ingredients but still comply with the labeling law because the GM content is below the applicable threshold.[14] Consumers who reject GM foods as a matter of principle will not actually know whether the foods they purchase or consume contain some GM, so the labeling will not enable them to avoid genetically modified foods altogether.[15] In addition, as a result of mistakes, trace contamination, or deliberate noncompliance, some other foods also not labeled as containing GM products inevitably contain some GM ingredients that should have triggered the labeling requirement, as empirical studies have already demonstrated.[16]

A further practical problem with the "right to know" rationale is that there is uncertainty and disagreement about where to draw the line between GM and non-GM foods, which further dilutes the potential for GM labels to enable individual choice. GM labeling advocates take inconsistent positions on whether foods such as cheese, beer, bread, and yogurt that are made using genetically engineered microbes are "GM," or whether products from animals fed GM feed should be labeled as GM.[17] As Alan McHughen succinctly summarizes the problem, "No matter what your position, GM labels fail to provide their intended raison d'être—informed choice."[18]

More broadly, any "right to know" cannot be absolute: "There is no prima facie case that consumers have the right to know everything through mandated labels or at any cost," writes Kalaitzandonakes.[19] Nor is the consumers' autonomy absolute in that it overrides every other consideration. As Peter Markie has noted, "Car dealers will promote their customers' autonomy by telling them when the same automobile can be purchased for less elsewhere or as part of an upcoming sale, assuming that the customers value paying the lowest price possible. Customers clearly do not have a right against dealers to be provided with this information, however."[20]

The list of information that consumers might be interested in having disclosed on their food labels is almost endless, including whether or not pesticides were used in production of the food, its insect and rodent droppings content, the labor practices of the food processor, or the soil conservation practices of the farmer.[21] For many of these factors, public support for disclosure may be stronger than for disclosure of genetic modification. For example, a higher proportion of the public would prefer labeling of pesticide content in foods than labeling for genetic modification.[22] Yet, for almost half a century, the FDA has consistently rejected any mandatory labeling of pesticide content in foods for both legal and practical reasons.[23] If every consumer desire for process-related information were honored, there would not be enough space on most food product labels to include it all.

The "right to know" rationale for GM labeling faces legal as well as practical problems. In striking down a Vermont law requiring milk producers to label milk produced from cows treated with the recombinant hormone bovine somatotrophin (rBST), the U.S. Court of Appeals for the Second Circuit held that mandatory labeling requirements based on a consumer's right or desire to know was an unwarranted intrusion on the constitutional rights of the dairy manufacturers:

> Although the Court is sympathetic to the Vermont consumers who wish to know which products may derive from [cows treated with the synthetic hormone rBST], their desire is insufficient to permit the State of Vermont to compel the dairy manufacturers to

speak against their will. Were consumer interest alone sufficient, there is no end to the information that states could require manufacturers to disclose about their production methods. . . . Absent, however, some indication that this information bears on a reasonable concern for human health or safety or some other sufficiently substantial governmental concern, the manufacturers cannot be compelled to disclose it.[24]

As discussed in chapter 2, a U.S. federal court has likewise already held that consumers' desire to know is not a legally sufficient rationale for the FDA to require companies to provide GM content information on their product labels.[25]

Finally, as will be discussed in more detail in chapter 8, consumers can already ensure that the foods they buy contain no intentionally added GM ingredients by selecting only foods that are certified organic or voluntarily labeled as non-GM.[26] Thus, any consumer "right to know" can already be satisfied by voluntary and market mechanisms, which avoid many of the costs and burdens of mandatory labeling requirements.

4

Consumer Choice

According to proponents of mandatory GM labels, consumers should have the choice of whether or not to consume GM foods, which purportedly can only be satisfied by mandatory GM labeling. For example, Greenpeace states that the purpose of mandatory labeling of GM food should be "to inform consumers about the production process and to allow an informed choice between genetically engineered and conventional food products."[1] Similarly, BEUC, the European Consumers' Organization, while stating that it is "not against these new [GM] products as such," and does not "suggest that consumers should not eat them for food safety reasons," advocates mandatory labeling on the ground that "the principle of consumer choice must be respected in the way in which these products are marketed."[2] The American Public Health Association likewise adopted a position statement in favor of GM labeling because such labeling "upholds and is consistent with the principle of consumer choice," adding that "any opposition to labeling based on findings that genetically modified food products are safe discounts issues of consumer choice and bioethical concerns."[3]

Yet, the empirical record is now clear that mandatory GM labeling thwarts, rather than promotes, consumer choice. Indeed, while many consumers no doubt support GM labeling based on a sincere belief that it would promote choice, the activists behind many of the pro-labeling campaigns have a very different agenda. They view mandatory labeling as the first step to excluding GM products from the market and denying consumers the choice of whether to buy them. Once GM products have been labeled, they can be specifically targeted for removal by either governmental regulation or by pressure tactics against grocery store chains, other retailers, food processors, and other participants in the food supply chain.

This is precisely what has happened in Europe and other jurisdictions that have adopted mandatory GM labeling requirements. Not content with the stringent, mandatory GM labeling and traceability scheme for which they successfully lobbied, European activist groups are now exploiting the very same labels that they justified on the grounds of consumer choice as a tool to achieve "an implicit market ban on GM food."[4]

For example, a survey of four major supermarkets in the Paris region of France found only two GM products available for sale.[5] In the United Kingdom, all major supermarket chains have now refused to stock any labeled GM products in response to pressure from the same groups that lobbied initially for GM labeling.[6] GM foods also disappeared from the shelves of Japanese grocery stores shortly after Japan imposed a mandatory labeling requirement.[7]

Following the launch of the European GM labeling requirement, Greenpeace announced that it would summon thousands of volunteers across Europe, whom it referred to as "gene detectives," to police grocery stores to ensure they were not stocking foods with GM labels.[8] As described in one report, Greenpeace local groups "send letters to the supermarket directors and the food processing companies, [and] organize rallies in front of supermarkets, using large poster[s] claiming that these supermarkets are 'contaminated with GM foods.'"[9] When a new Swedish beer became the first European food put on the market with the new "genetically modified" label required by the EU rules, "Greenpeace responded by shadowing the beer's first delivery trucks through the streets of Copenhagen and pressuring store owners into barring the beer from their shelves."[10] According to the Greenpeace protest leader, "We stayed up all night printing materials to hand out at the stores and arranging chase cars, but it was worth it."[11] This type of protest action creates a first-mover disadvantage in which any food supplier or retailer that attempted to break the implicit ban on GM foods would be instantly targeted for intense opposition and controversy, deterring any such sales.[12] The GM label has been transformed into a scarlet letter that enables these anti-choice tactics and campaigns.

One Greenpeace leader boasted about the group's concerted campaign to prevent European consumers from having a choice of buying GM products:

> The market is practically free of products containing GMOs. This
> is a great success for consumers. Their rejection of GMOs in food
> has made major food producers and retailers ensure that their
> shelves are free of modified products.[13]

So much for giving consumers a choice. These actions by activists to prevent consumers from choosing GM foods are starkly at odds with the
pro–consumer choice rhetoric used to justify GM labeling in Europe and
elsewhere. The result has been that European consumers are denied the
right to choose whether or not to purchase GM foods.

Activists in the United States are pursuing a similar one-two punch of
first trying to get GM foods labeled by mandatory government regulations,
followed by de facto bans of such products by pressure tactics that target
labeled GM products. For example, proponents of mandatory GM labeling

> make no secret that mandatory labeling is not their final goal.
> They admit that they support a moratorium or ban on GM crops,
> and that they are planning to lobby the Environmental Protec-
> tion Agency to get the moratorium passed. Yet their strategic
> focus is placed on mandatory labeling. The reason is that they
> have learned from the consequences in the EU of its mandatory
> labeling requirement. GM food resistance among environmental
> groups and consumers in the EU, with mandatory labeling as a
> tool, has triggered a de facto moratorium.[14]

Along the same lines, Congressman Dennis Kucinich, the leading proponent of mandatory GM labeling in the U.S. Congress, has stated, "I think
if we were to come out immediately and say they [GM foods] should be
banned, I'm not quite sure if we could get the kind of constituency moving
forward at this moment on that issue. I think the issue of labeling could
achieve that in the short-term."[15]

Thus, anti-GM activists and their political supporters use mandatory
GM labeling as a "Trojan horse" to achieve their true purpose of banning
GM foods:

> Most of the environmental activists who are opposed to GM
> foods strongly support mandatory labeling policies. Why would

they do so if they knew that it would insure a place for GM food at the retail level? To the contrary, these groups may be using mandatory labeling as a type of Trojan horse: they support mandatory labeling for the sake of consumer choice, knowing full well that this policy will lead to no choice in practice. Moreover, even if there are some products that are labeled as a result, the products can be easily targeted by the activists.[16]

It is important to note that the activists seeking to use mandatory GM labels as a tool to ban GM foods are focusing their efforts on companies, not consumers.[17] Polls show that many consumers who support GM labeling would also be willing to purchase GM-labeled products. For example, a survey by the Center for Science in the Public Interest found that 40 percent of consumers in a national telephone poll of randomly selected U.S. adults would potentially be willing to purchase labeled GM foods if given the choice between a GM product and an equivalent non-GM product, with 38 percent indifferent between the two products and 8 percent preferring the GM product.[18] Attempts by activist groups to persuade consumers to exercise their market choices and refrain from purchasing GM labeled foods would be a legitimate, pro-democratic, and pro-market activity, provided the arguments and information they used were credible. Such activities would be consistent with free markets and the exercise of informed consumer choice. The activists seeking to ban GM foods are not, however, willing to rely on consumer choice, because they know that many consumers will choose to purchase GM foods. As the leader of Greenpeace's campaign to block the sales of GM foods in Europe admitted, "If consumers start buying [GM foods] and get used to it, we will lose."[19] There would be no need to pressure food producers and retailers against providing GM foods if no consumers would buy them—the market itself would ensure that such unpopular products were not available.

Thus, rather than legitimately trying to influence consumer choice, these organizations have focused their efforts on depriving consumers of the opportunity to make a choice by targeting food processors and retailers. Given their low profit margins and the relatively small share of the final product represented by GM ingredients in most processed foods, such companies are likely to capitulate to protestors to avoid losing any segment of their market comprising those who may boycott the stores and create bad publicity harmful to overall sales.[20] The result, as shown by the outcome in Europe and elsewhere, will be that companies will substitute non-GM ingredients for GM content to avoid having to label their products. Any company that then tries to introduce a food product with GM ingredients will become a lightening rod of controversy, further deterring any attempt to make GM products available to consumers.

The outcome of these dynamics will be a de facto ban on GM products, whereby the extreme views of a vocal minority deprive the rest of the population of a choice that will afford them the benefits of biotechnology, including consumers in developing countries who may benefit most from its continued development.[21] As the United Nations Development Report noted in 2001, "Transgenics offer the hope of crops with higher yields, pest- and drought-resistant properties and superior nutritional characteristics—especially for farmers in ecological zones left behind by the green revolution."[22] Thus, "the current debate in Europe and the U.S. over genetically modified crops mostly ignores the concerns and needs of the developing world"[23] and tends to be driven by the views of Western consumers, "who do not face food shortages or nutritional deficiencies, or work in the fields."[24]

5

Public Opinion

Another argument used to support mandatory GM labeling is that public opinion overwhelmingly supports GM labeling. According to advocates, in a democratic nation this fact alone is sufficient to justify regulations imposing such a requirement. For example, in its position paper in favor of mandatory GM food labeling, the Consumers Union declares that "since labeling laws are created to meet consumer needs, consumer opinion should be respected."[1] Similarly, two supporters of mandatory labeling contend, "In the United States, an overwhelming majority of citizens believe that GM foods should be labeled as such; the same is true in Europe. Thus, respecting citizen autonomy also supports positive labeling."[2]

To be sure, many public opinion polls appear to demonstrate overwhelming public support for GM labeling. Polls by various media entities and policy organizations have consistently found that 75 percent or more of the public, when asked whether they favor GM food labeling, answer in the affirmative.[3] For example, a 2002 poll commissioned by the Center for Food Policy found that 88.4 percent of surveyed adult U.S. voters strongly or somewhat agreed that the federal government should require labels on all genetically engineered food products,[4] and a 2004 poll by Rutgers' Food Policy Institute found that 89 percent of respondents supported labeling of GM foods.[5] In these and similar polls, it is important to note that no mention was made of the costs associated with a mandatory labeling program.

Putting aside the issue of whether majority public opinion is automatically sufficient to dictate public policy, especially concerning a scientifically complex issue about which public knowledge and understanding are limited, the public opinion rationale fails to stand up to deeper scrutiny. There are several problems with relying on these polling results.

First, the polls that ask people whether they would prefer GM foods to be labeled usually do not measure the depth or sophistication of the views of the respondents. In fact, other survey formats strongly indicate that most people do not feel strongly about the labeling of GM foods, notwithstanding the magnitude of the percentage who claim they support it when specifically asked. For example, if, instead of expressly asking people whether they support GM labeling, the pollster instead asks respondents what additional information they would like on food labels without giving them answers to choose from, fewer than 1 percent identify biotechnology or genetic modification as a concern they want added to the label.[6]

Other survey evidence further suggests that consumer support for mandatory GM labeling is weak. When told they could only add one additional piece of information to food labels from a list of possible items, almost twice as many respondents (31 percent versus 17 percent) chose to include labeling on trace amounts of pesticide present over disclosure that the food was genetically engineered.[7] This is particularly significant given that one of the benefits of GM foods is to reduce pesticide use. Another survey question described the FDA's policy of not requiring special labeling for GM foods unless the modification introduces an allergen or substantially changes the food's nutritional content. Only 13 percent of consumers strongly or somewhat opposed the FDA's policy, while 60 percent strongly or somewhat supported it.[8]

Some evidence also suggests that public support for mandatory GM labeling is often confused and not consistent with either scientific knowledge or the purported rationales for it. For example, in a study in the United Kingdom that found that 75 percent of consumers supported GM labeling, the primary rationale that citizens gave for wanting such labeling was to provide a warning on health risks.[9] Yet, as discussed above, the EU and other governments that have adopted mandatory GM labeling have expressly disavowed any health-risk warning rationale. Thus, public support is inconsistent not only with scientific knowledge but also with any governmental justification for mandatory labeling.

A recent study conducted in Canada examining what people actually do, rather than what they say they would do, also demonstrated a lack of serious interest in GM labels.[10] Women at a shopping center were asked to participate in a survey that they were told was evaluating consumer response to a new breakfast cereal. The subjects in the study were then given a box of the cereal and a sample and asked to respond to a short questionnaire. Some of the women were given a cereal box that had no information on GM content, others were given a box that stated GM ingredients were present, and still others were given a box that affirmatively stated no GM ingredients were present. There were no significant differences in the subjects' interest in purchasing the cereal. The results led the study author to conclude that "if a GM label provides no useful information, there are serious questions about its value."[11]

Another study conducted in France, where public sentiment against GM foods is among the strongest in the world, adds further evidence that public demands for labeling may be weak.[12] In this study, French consumers were given two chocolate bars that were identical except that one was labeled as containing genetically engineered corn. The subjects were asked to examine the two products in their wrappers for three minutes and then indicate how much they were willing to pay for each chocolate bar. There was no difference in the average value the subjects were willing to pay for the GM-labeled chocolate bar as opposed to the unlabeled bar. This result suggested that a GM label would have little real-world impact, because most consumers do not spend three minutes examining the labels of most food products they buy, and thus would presumably ignore the GM label.

In the next stage of the study, the list of ingredients (which included the GM label) for each product was magnified and projected on an overhead screen, and the subjects were invited to read the list of ingredients. Only in this context, when their attention was specifically directed to the text that included the GM label, did the consumers' average willingness to pay for the GM-labeled chocolate bar decrease relative to the unlabeled bar, and even then only by a modest 27.3 percent. The authors appropriately entitled their published paper, "Do Consumers Not Care About Biotech Foods or Do They Just Not Read the Labels?" Regardless of which answer is correct, the results further indicate that the alleged overwhelming public demand for GM labeling is more suggestive and theoretical than deeply felt and readily recalled. Other studies find a similar lack of genuine consumer interest in GM labels. For example, in a study that assessed consumers' interest in eight different characteristics of a snack food, GM content was the least important.[13]

Some limited empirical data are now available evaluating consumers' real-world food purchasing preferences, as opposed to preferences measured in simulated or hypothetical study settings. These data show that people's stated preferences in a survey in support of GM labeling are not matched by actual purchasing decisions in the real world.[14] For example, one recent study demonstrated that, in the aggregate, consumers in the Netherlands did not appreciably change their food-purchasing behavior after GM-containing foods were labeled.[15] Studies in China similarly found only a minor 2–4 percent short-term decline in sales of GM cooking oil after mandatory labels were enforced.[16] Moreover, this small impact of labeling was restricted exclusively to upper-income consumers, whereas lower-income shoppers were not at all affected.[17]

Similarly, a large study funded by the EU of real-life consumer behavior toward GM foods in ten EU nations observed:

> Whatever they may have said in response to questions, most shoppers did not actively avoid GM-products, suggesting they were not greatly concerned with the GM issue. Moreover, it is clear that, as far as buying GM-foods is concerned, the way people respond to prompting via questionnaires and polls is by itself not a reliable guide to what they will buy in a grocery store.[18]

The study concluded:

> Overall, people seem not to be able to recognize GM-food in spite of the labelling requirements. But this does not appear to be a problem as people . . . in general are not careful to avoid these products, a conclusion supported by the scant attention paid to labels.[19]

This largest study to date of actual consumer behavior in the stores toward GM foods is particularly significant, given that it was funded by the very government entity that has imposed the world's most stringent GM labeling requirements, and that it studied the population (that is, the EU public) that allegedly is most adamantly in support of GM labeling.

Yet, more confirmation that the demand for mandatory GM labeling is actually rather weak comes from Oregon Ballot Measure 27 of 2002, which proposed to require labeling of all genetically engineered foods. The measure failed overwhelmingly, with over 70 percent of voters rejecting mandatory labeling.[20] Initial polls when the referendum was placed on the ballot showed a 20 percent lead for the "yes" side, but as the public learned more about the costs and problems of GM labeling, public opinion swayed heavily against it.

Taken together, these results suggest that the alleged support for GM labeling is superficial. If asked specifically whether they would like GM labeling, people generally reply affirmatively, but the other studies summarized above show that this sentiment is not a strongly held or considered opinion, and it may be nonexistent in real-life purchasing decisions or when provided with more context, such as the existing regulatory approach to U.S. food labeling.

Perhaps even more important, the polls asking the public whether they support GM labeling are generally structurally flawed. If pollsters were to ask citizens whether they would like a new Porsche, the vast majority would most likely answer yes, much as a large majority say they would rather have GM labeling than not. Yet, if you were to ask people whether they would like a new Porsche but would have to pay to get it, many more people would no longer answer affirmatively. In the same way, while the vast majority of people say they would support GM labeling if no costs are mentioned or imposed, the result is very different if people are asked to pay for the additional costs associated with GM labeling.[21] As one former supporter of mandatory GM labeling who now opposes such a requirement has written, "it is facile and misleading" to conclude that people want GM labeling from surveys that do not disclose the burdens and costs of such requirements. "People need to know the consequences of policies" to make meaningful decisions on whether or not to support them.[22]

As will be discussed in chapter 7, mandatory labeling of GM foods, and the segregation of the food supply system required to implement such a labeling scheme, impose significant costs on farmers, distributors, food processors, and retailers, most of which would presumably be passed on to consumers in higher food prices.[23] These costs would include not only establishing separate collection, storage, transportation, and processing chains for GM and non-GM foods, but also the various administrative, paperwork, testing, and liability costs that would be imposed by a mandatory labeling requirement.[24]

The previously mentioned 2001 public opinion poll by the Center for Science in the Public Interest found that 77 percent of the public would not be willing to pay more than $50 per year per household for GM labeling, with 44 percent of respondents not willing to pay anything extra.[25] Only 12 percent of Americans were willing to pay $250 per household for such labeling. Even among the people who supported mandatory labeling of GM foods, 56 percent would pay nothing or only $10 per year for it. In other words, given that the costs per household of a mandatory GM labeling scheme would easily exceed $10 per year under virtually all cost estimates of such a program, a majority of consumers oppose mandatory GM labeling if they are required to pay for it, which at least indirectly will inevitably be the case.

Other contingent valuation surveys show that while some consumers are willing to pay significantly more for their food to avoid GM ingredients, many others—in most studies the majority of respondents—are not willing to pay the extra costs that GM labeling would impose.[26] One such study found that the majority (between 52 percent and 70 percent, depending on the survey methodology used) of U.S. consumers were either unwilling or uncertain about their willingness to pay a premium to avoid genetically modified breakfast cereal.[27] On average, American consumers were willing to pay only a modest premium (10–12 percent) to avoid GM foods, although U.K. consumers were willing to pay a somewhat higher premium (19–35 percent). Given that a majority of Americans did not indicate a willingness to pay extra to avoid GM foods, the authors concluded that "mandatory labeling could be a serious overregulation that imposes greater costs on the entire public if a significant segment of the population does not have a preference for non-biotech foods."[28] True willingness to pay for GM labeling is almost certainly even lower than estimated in this and other studies using similar surveys, since the contingent-value methodology used tends to overestimate consumer willingness to pay due to hypothetical bias, in which consumers' estimates of how much they are willing to pay in an imaginary exercise is significantly higher than they would actually pay with their own money in the real world.[29]

Another study involved conducting a contingent-value survey of shoppers in three locations in Colorado to determine how much they would be willing to pay for a GM labeling scheme.[30] The study found that the mean willingness to pay (WTP) for mandatory GM labeling was between $81 and $134 per household (depending on the statistical model used), amounts that, the authors observed, were well below the estimated costs of actually implementing such a labeling scheme. Moreover, as the study authors acknowledged, the WTP values they reported were probably overestimates because only subjects who supported a mandatory or voluntary GM labeling scheme were enrolled in the study. The authors concluded that "only a small proportion of the population" would be willing to pay the costs associated with a mandatory GM labeling program.[31]

Other studies have likewise found only a modest willingness to pay for GM labeling that likely would not outweigh the actual costs of a labeling and segregation requirement. A survey of U.S. consumers found that a label on cornflakes stating that the product "contains genetically modified corn" would reduce the price consumers would pay for that product on average by 6.5 percent, whereas a label that the product "may contain genetically modified corn" would only reduce willingness to pay by 1 percent.[32] Another study found that only 35–41 percent (depending on the product) were willing to pay any extra price for a non-GM versus a GM version of the food product at issue.[33] Although 58 percent of participants were willing to pay more for a non-GM version of at least one of the three food items in the survey, the fact that considerably fewer than 50 percent were willing to pay extra for any specific product to be non-GM suggests that labeling of any (or each) product would be contrary to majority opinion.

In conclusion, while implementing mandatory GM labeling is often portrayed as giving the people what they want and consistent with overwhelming public opinion, more careful analysis reveals that such a labeling program would actually be contrary to the stated and revealed preferences of most of the population. In other words, rather than supporting mandatory GM labeling, public opinion, when surveyed in a more realistic and holistic manner, actually weighs against it.

6

Tracking and Surveillance Applications

A final rationale often cited as supporting the need for mandatory GM labeling is that such labels could be useful for tracking the origins and contents of food with respect to whether they were genetically modified. This could allegedly serve a variety of purposes, such as monitoring long-term health problems, identifying at-risk products and consumers if a problem should arise, and allowing people of specific religious faiths to adhere to appropriate dietary restrictions. As discussed below, none of these purported rationales stands up to critical scrutiny.

Health Monitoring and Product Surveillance

Some advocates of mandatory GM labels argue that such labeling would enable monitoring and detection of any long-term health risks associated with GM foods.[1] For example, the *San Francisco Chronicle* reported that "a lack of labels makes it difficult to track an increase in allergic reactions or some other pattern of health problems to a genetically engineered ingredient or food."[2] A related potential traceability benefit of mandatory GM labeling would be to help identify at-risk products and consumers if a health problem were to emerge for one or more GM products on the market. According to this line of reasoning, if a GM product were to prove harmful, the mandatory labels would help identify individuals who had consumed that product, who could then be monitored and treated, if necessary, for any adverse health effects. Moreover, any remaining product on the market could be identified and recalled. Finally, a related claimed benefit of tracking GM ingredients would be to use the mandatory labels to assign responsibility and liability to specific companies that had produced harmful GM products. One of the environmental movement's most vocal *supporters* of the benefits of biotech crops, Jason Clay of the World Wildlife Fund/U.S., states this rationale as follows:

> Without labeling it is impossible to tell which products contain GMOs, thus minimizing liability exposure starting at the retail level, including manufacturers, refiners/processors and the major grain trading companies as well. In short, when corporations do not know there are genetically modified ingredients in their products, they have plausible deniability if ever questioned by consumers. This explains why efforts to block GM labeling for genetically modified ingredients are in the United States, where consumers are more litigious.[3]

An example often cited to support the traceability benefits of mandatory GM labeling is a 1989 incident in which lot-based traceability was used to impose a multi-billion-dollar liability on a manufacturer who sold an animal feed ingredient (l-tryptophan) produced in genetically engineered microorganisms, which natural food companies diverted to unlabeled "health food" uses. Specifically, plaintiffs alleged that the genetically modified bacterium used in production of the amino acid l-tryptophan caused "eosinophilia myalgia syndrome" (EMS), an autoimmune-type illness, in several thousand plaintiffs, resulting in thirty-seven deaths. The resulting l-tryptophan mass-tort litigation demonstrated that those manufacturers who did not have lot-based traceability could hide behind deniability, while the major manufacturer (Showa Denko KK) was subjected to significant traceback liability, reported in the press as reaching several billion dollars.[4]

A number of contaminants may have acted in concert to cause EMS in this incident,[5] and this uncertainty makes it difficult to link the harm, as activists like to do, to the process of genetic engineering.[6] In the "litigious" U.S. court system, however, the lack of an identifiable cause did not stop a California jury from awarding $1 million to a woman who was warned by the FDA not to take this recalled product.[7] Approximately 1,600 other claims were settled, providing compensation in spite of the uncertain conclusions reached after extensive lot-based tracing back and examination of impurities in the products.

This idea that GM labels would have aided health monitoring and traceability on products sold with GM-derived l-tryptophan, or biotech inputs generally, does not stand up to scrutiny. Having a generic "GM" label would not have led to discovery of those manufacturers of l-tryptophan that did not have traceability systems in place. Even if a particular GM product should, for the sake of argument, subsequently turn out to present a significant health risk, it is hard to see how generic GM labels would expedite a health-related investigation, when the standard of proof in law or science requires specific (for example, lot-based) traceability to investigate the cause of particular adverse health events. Every jurisdiction that has mandated GM labeling has required *generic* label language, such as "This product contains genetically modified ingredients," that provides no traceability to source. At most, the label might identify the commodity crop that was genetically modified (for instance, corn or soybean),[8] but it says nothing about the type of genetic modification, the engineered trait, or the specific cultivar used in a specific product. It could be any GM input, for all consumers or health investigators know. This generic warning about a single process used in numerous crops gives manufacturers the same level of plausible deniability as no label at all, as a practical matter. In general, more specific information provided by product-specific traceability would be needed to be of any use to a retrospective safety study, current surveillance, or identification of potentially affected individuals.[9]

The generic GM label would only be potentially useful if all, or nearly all, GM foods shared some common toxicity. If this proved to be the case, a retrospective recall would likely have to use genetic testing of foods to remove the entire range of GM inputs from the shelves, since the labels at one tolerance (0.9 percent) would not cover an allergen having an effect at very low levels. Moreover, in nations where almost all residents have consumed some corn- or soy-based foods containing genetically modified ingredients on multiple occasions, any consumers who reported having seen a GM label on their food would simply tell us what we already know— that they, like almost everyone else in their community, have consumed a wide variety of GM foods.[10] Moreover, a voluntary non-GMO labeling scheme would work as well as, if not better than, mandatory GM labeling to create a non-exposed "control" group to compare and follow in long-term studies of possible health effects.

Mandatory labeling of GM foods to promote traceability would not only be ineffective and unnecessary to achieve the stated objectives of protecting human health; it would also be unfair and scientifically unsupported. As discussed in chapter 1, virtually all foods use crops that have been "genetically modified" over time, whether by modern biotechnology, chemical or nuclear mutagenesis, or selective breeding. As a result, there is broad scientific consensus that GM foods are inherently no more risky or likely to cause illness than any other type of food. Thus, a requirement to label GM foods but not other foods that are also genetically modified, via mutagenesis or other processes, for the purpose of tracking any potential health problems is inherently arbitrary and lacks any scientific justification.[11]

In sum, the premise that GM foods should be singled out for generic process labeling to serve public health investigational purposes is not scientifically credible, nor does it serve any corporate liability-prevention strategy.

Cultural and Religious Dietary Restrictions

Another related tracking argument often advanced for requiring GM food labels is that they are necessary to help people from various religious and cultural groups to observe dietary laws and customs.[12] Most Jewish denominations, for example, refrain from eating pork, devout Catholics abstain from eating red meat on Fridays, and some Buddhists adhere to a strict vegan diet.[13] Without GM food labeling, its proponents argue, people might unknowingly eat foods that violate their religious practices.[14]

There are several problems with this argument. First, it is implicitly premised on a fallacy that a gene from one species somehow confers many of the properties and even the essence of that species when it is transferred to another. To the contrary, a gene transferred from another species is usually chemically similar to an existing gene in the modified species, differing only in a few DNA base pairs that affect the folding and function of the resulting protein. So, if a gene from a fish is used to modify a tomato (the product of which, despite much sensationalist media coverage, is not commercially available), the small chemical change in the DNA does not transfer any fish-like properties to the tomato. It does not taste like a fish, it does not smell like a fish, and it doesn't in any way look like a fish. In fact, it has no fish properties whatsoever except a slightly different version of an exist-ing protein. As Henry Miller has written, "Parts of the nucleic acid sequence of *Escherichia coli* are identical to that of organisms such as oilseed rape, amphibians, birds, grasses, and mammals—including humans. Such find-ings put in doubt the value of assigning genes to a particular species."[15]

Second, at least at this time, no commercially available GM foods are the product of gene transfers that could possibly offend the dietary practices of any recognized religion.[16] In fact, many of the major religions have publicly announced that their members may eat GM foods, including the Jewish,[17] Catholic,[18] and Islamic[19] faiths.

Third, even if such foods are developed in the future, religious people who seek certain diets, such as kosher, already have private systems in place to ensure the purity of their foods, and those private systems would presumably incorporate prohibitions on certain gene transfers (if any) that may violate the relevant dietary codes. For example, just as kosher food producers contractually require their suppliers to certify that their ingredi-ents comply with kosher requirements, a food producer who wanted to ensure that its products contained no GM to satisfy religious or other pref-erences would likewise require its suppliers to use ingredients that were traced to non-GM inputs.

Fourth, a U.S. federal district court has already evaluated the claim that GM labeling is necessary to protect religious practices and found the argu-ment to be without merit—the lack of GM labeling, the court ruled, amounted to no more than a "potential inconvenience" and certainly not a significant burden on any established religious practice.[20]

Finally, as one religious leader wrote, if we require mandatory GM labeling of foods to satisfy religious preferences, "we might soon run out of space on many food products for legible labeling as various minority groups—religious and lifestyle—claimed the statutory right to their par-ticular labeling requirements."[21]

***

To conclude, there is no valid tracking or surveillance justification that com-pels mandatory GM labeling, whether it be to research or track potential health impacts associated with GM foods, to enable compliance with religious or cultural dietary practices, or for any other purpose. As the American Medical Association concluded in its 2000 position paper on GM foods, "There is no scientific justification for special labeling of genetically modified foods, as a class."[22]

PART III

Arguments against Mandatory GM Labeling

7

Costs and Burdens of Mandatory GM Labeling

Aside from the lack of a legitimate purpose for it, another consideration weighing against mandatory GM labeling is the substantial cost of such a requirement. This chapter summarizes the economic costs, trade disruption, and other burdens resulting from mandatory GM food labeling regimes. These are not hypothetical, but are increasingly being experienced today across the globe as a result of mandatory GM labeling laws. In particular, mandatory labeling in Europe and Asia is imposing significant economic and opportunity costs without commensurate benefits, over and above the global disruptions being triggered by general opposition to biotechnology crops. Four types of costs, disruptions, and burdens are discussed below:

- the direct costs of testing and segregation of GM products to comply with mandatory labeling requirements;

- economic distortion of markets resulting in decisions to forgo GM products notwithstanding the benefits and market demand for such products;

- food shipment disruptions; and

- consumer confusion.

Costs of Testing and Segregation

The actual physical label required on a GM-containing product is, by itself, relatively inexpensive, involving the costs for designing and printing it; for multinationals trading in many overseas markets, however, the requirement may involve the cost of over forty different labels, each of which must be tracked to ensure that a product with the appropriate label is sent to the correct market. The product testing and segregation necessary to ensure compliance with a mandatory GM labeling requirement are, however, much more expensive and burdensome. The food production and distribution system in the United States does not easily accommodate segregation of GM crops and product from their non-GM counterparts. From the farm equipment used to harvest crops, to the trucks used to bring the crops from the farm to the market, to the grain elevators used to store the crops, to the ships, trucks, train cars, and other containers used to transport the grains, to the processing and production facilities used to process the raw materials, to the packaging and distribution chains used to bring the final product to market, GM and non-GM inputs are typically mixed together.

To comply with a mandatory GM labeling scheme, this entire food supply system, from "farm to fork," will need to be duplicated and kept separate to ensure segregation of GM from non-GM product.[1] Many parts of the distribution system will need to be regularly emptied and cleaned to prevent unwanted commingling of crops in machinery or containers used in storage or transport; in some instances, the capital expense of an entire additional duplicate system for storage and transport must be installed. Finally, to ensure compliance with the labeling requirement, product streams will need to be tested regularly at various points along the supply chain to check for such contamination. As one description summarized the challenge:

> Many of the grain elevators and other storage depots that farmers bring their harvests to don't have multiple bins or the capacity needed to keep engineered and non-engineered varieties apart. . . . Moreover, elevator operators would have to clean their equipment between batches to prevent any carryover of engineered varieties into conventional ones—a difficult job that would cost the company time and wages. And what if some contamination occurred? Who would be responsible? . . . It would be very easy to get a truck mixed up. . . . And if you contaminate [the distributor's] supply, there's a potential for liability.[2]

The actual costs of a GM labeling and segregation system will depend on the parameters of the specific labeling requirements, such as the threshold level (that is, tolerance) and the traceability requirements (if any) and the rigor of the enforcement and certification process, as well as characteristics of the relevant food distribution system and market.[3] Not surprisingly, then, given the many factors that can affect them, cost estimates vary significantly and are subject to considerable uncertainty. Nevertheless, a GM labeling and segregation system would unquestionably involve significant costs and burdens and would, in essence, impose a new tax on farmers, food processors, distributors, retailers, and, ultimately, the consumer.[4]

One often-cited cost estimate for mandatory GM labeling was provided in a study by the accounting firm KPMG Consulting, commissioned by the Australian and New Zealand governments, which found that such a requirement would result in reduced profits for food companies and increases in consumer prices for foods ranging from 0.5–15 percent.[5] Another study by KPMG on mandatory GM labeling, this time in Canada, projected an increase in the cost of all subject processed foods of 9–10 percent.[6] An analysis of the costs of a segregated food chain to separate GM and non-GM canola under a voluntary labeling scheme estimated that such an identity-preservation system would increase relevant food costs by 13–15 percent.[7] As one set of economic researchers summarized the evidence, "One conclusion seems apparent: Implementing a labeling policy on GM foods is costly and involves uncertain effects on firms, consumers, and the industry."[8]

The EU imposes additional cost burdens in its GM labeling scheme by not only requiring segregation and labeling, but also by imposing an accompanying traceability requirement. Each link in the distribution chain from farm to fork for each ingredient in the final food product must transfer documentation of GM status from the previous and to the next link in the chain. Documentation must also be retained for five years at each stage of the chain of supply, and food manufacturers and exporters are responsible for preparing documents describing the GM content of any product they sell or buy. The objective of this traceability directive is to ensure that no product made "from" GM crops or ingredients reaches the market without a GM label.

These tracking and paperwork requirements impose significant additional costs on GM suppliers and processors that are not imposed on producers of non-GM foods, and they create the potential for legal and economic risks if undocumented genetic modifications are found in low levels in the food or feed. Indeed, empirical cost estimates of the EU labeling and traceability requirements are not available because, as discussed in the next section, almost all EU farmers, food processors, and food retailers have concluded that they are too burdensome to comply with, making it more cost-effective to avoid GM inputs.

In discussing the costs of a mandatory GM labeling program, it bears mention that the burden of these costs would be distributed regressively. In other words, the costs of mandatory GM labeling would fall disproportionately on low-income consumers, who spend a greater proportion of their available income on food.[9] Thus, it is not only the magnitude of the cost burden but also the distribution of those costs that create concerns about a mandatory GM labeling regime.

Market Distortions

Among the most profound and immediate impacts of mandatory GM food labeling laws may be the market distortions that will force exclusion of GM foods from the market, notwithstanding the considerable benefits and market demand associated with such products.[10] For example, as discussed above, the EU labeling and traceability requirements are currently imposing minimal direct costs, but significant price increases for large quantities of non-GM corn and soybeans imported from non-U.S. sources. The GM labeling law effectively keeps GM foods from the European market, given the prohibitive costs and burdens of compliance. As a result, few, if any, food products are incurring the costs of complying with the burdensome EU labeling and traceability requirements. Because the food industry operates on generally small profit margins, any additional costs or restrictions imposed by mandatory GM labels will create compelling financial pressures for farmers, food processors, and retailers to forgo GM products.[11] Thus, the most important societal cost imposed by mandatory GM labeling in the EU and elsewhere is to force large-scale market substitution of GM source material for reasons unrelated to the merits or benefits of GM products.

The market distortions imposed by mandatory GM labeling and trace-ability requirements are particularly acute when the labeling laws set exceedingly low tolerances, such as the 0.9 percent threshold enforced by the EU. These low thresholds for trace GM crops are so difficult and expensive to test for in a consistent and reliable manner that food manufacturers would not normally agree to meet them in the marketplace and, therefore, will seek non-GM alternatives.

For example, the EU's strict labeling tolerance is below international seed standards that start at 1 percent for genetic purity and have never, in the history of seed certification, delivered seed to a lower certified standard.[12] With most of the certified seed sold in North America and other biotech-producing production centers having warranties of genetic purity at 1 percent or greater, this presents a challenge for food and feed manufacturers who need large quantities of commodities transported to them from those locations. The EU's requirements demand genetic purity levels that the international agricultural seed production system cannot deliver.[13] With a more reasonable tolerance of 5 percent, such as that imposed by some Asian nations, U.S. exporters of non-GM soybean and corn thrive—whereas, at lower tolerances, the higher cost and risk of scientifically inevitable trade disruption chill the development of export markets.

Mandatory labeling requirements in other parts of the world have disrupted trade with the United States, particularly with respect to U.S. exports of corn, canola, or soybeans. Food companies reacted to such requirements by substituting non-GM inputs to avoid the high cost associated with labeling, the increased potential for inadvertent noncompliance, and the risk of losing a few percentage points of market share. Accordingly, the adoption of the GM label requirements immediately caused a steep reduction in the use of biotech inputs in processed food products exported to the EU and Asia. For example, Japan's largest maker of soybean protein food products, along with its three largest beer brewers, all declared that they would stop using any genetically modified ingredients after implementation of the country's GM labeling requirement.[14]

Similarly, when the EU tightened its GM labeling requirements in 2004 to include products made "from" GM products even if they lack detectable DNA or protein, U.S. exports of soybeans to Europe fell precipitously, even though all U.S. growers were using an EU-approved biotech Roundup

Ready soybean.[15] The American Soybean Association reported a drop of 65 percent in exports of soybean products to the EU, from $2.5 billion to $874 million per year, between 1997, when the initial less-burdensome GM labeling rules went into effect, and 2004, when the more stringent EU traceability and labeling requirements took effect.[16] This market dislocation has not only hurt U.S. farmers and food exporters, but has also threatened the viability of the EU animal feed industry, which has lost its primary supply source.[17] A recent analysis by the EU's Agricultural Directorate concluded that the EU's "zero tolerance" policy for unauthorized GM foods is causing a major feed shortage in the EU that will only get worse as new GM products are approved in exporting nations and could result, as a worst-case scenario, in a mass slaughter of livestock in Europe.[18]

Furthermore, the EU's GM labeling requirements compel less-developed nations that export agricultural products to adopt similar policies, if the supply chain is to meet the strict labeling standards.[19] In particular, if a developing nation begins to enforce GM labeling requirements strictly, it will be forced to choose between producing only non-GM crops or producing both GM and non-GM products and instituting expensive segregation and dual processing streams (one for GM, one for non-GM), along with burdensome traceability and recordkeeping obligations. To minimize costs and comply with the EU requirements, the developing nation will be forced to choose the first option and prohibit GM crops, even though it will lose whatever benefits it might otherwise have obtained from them.[20]

It is an axiom of international trade that multinationals adhere, for efficiency's sake, to the strictest standard imposed worldwide, so as to have a product that can be sold in as many markets as possible. The EU's stringent GM traceability and labeling law acts as a de facto reversal of regulatory approvals of GM foods and feeds, imposing harsh market distortions against GM crops in developing and developed nations that export their products to EU nations.

Shipping Disruption Incidents

Another "cost" imposed by mandatory GM labeling is the disruption that inevitably occurs whenever some nonlabeled GM product is discovered in a food shipment. As noted previously, the EU's labeling and traceability requirements that took effect in 2004 require that each separate GM crop variety be traced throughout the feed production process. Thus, if GM "contamination" is found in a food product, potential liability may apply up the distribution chain, and, perhaps even more damaging, the producing company and/or country may face a blockage of further shipments of its products.

A recent example of such a disruption resulted from the discovery that a low level of an unapproved GM rice strain ("Liberty Link") being developed by Bayer CropScience was present in the U.S. rice supply. Expert scientific bodies in the United States, the EU, and elsewhere concluded that the presence of low amounts of this rice strain presented no risks to human health, yet the discovery resulted in European and Asian refusal to accept U.S. rice imports.[21] This incident resulted in hundreds of millions of dollars of losses to U.S. farmers and food companies because of noncompliance with legal technicalities, including GM labeling requirements in European and Asian nations, even though no risks to humans or the environment were involved. The economic fallout was not limited to the United States, as EU rice millers who rely on American rice imports also suffered substantial losses, which, according to one report, "push[ed] the average EU rice miller into debt."[22]

A series of lawsuits has resulted to try to determine who should bear these economic losses. For example, in August 2007, a German food company (Rickmers Reismuehle GmbH) sued Riceland, a U.S. growers' cooperative, and an Arkansas mill for its costs associated with the recall in Europe of the unapproved Liberty Link rice found in a "non-GM" rice shipment.[23] Similarly, a coalition of U.S. rice producers has brought a consolidated series of cases against Bayer seeking compensation for their substantial economic losses.[24]

The EU's strict thresholds for GM contamination are particularly prone to creating such disruptions. While the EU's GM labeling law sets a very strict 0.9 percent tolerance for inadvertent, but otherwise authorized, GM content, an even tighter standard (effectively zero tolerance) applies to *know-able* or unauthorized GM content, which the EU has also construed very strictly. For example, in July 2005, EU enforcers threatened to take action against a German breakfast cereal manufacturer that used soy ingredients testing at 0.6 percent and 0.7 percent GM content. Since the government's tests showed a series of positive findings for the presence of GM ingredients, they concluded that the "contamination" was not necessarily "technically unavoidable" under the GM labeling law. The company's quality management files revealed a history of GM tests ranging from 0.1–0.4 percent, which showed that the cereal company "knowingly" used a soy ingredient that contained GM content—which could not therefore be truly "inadvertent." Regulators emphasized that an operator who knowingly uses GM ingredients in food production must verify that it was technically unavoidable. Unless the company can prove that no equivalent ingredient at less than 0.1 percent GM is available on the market, it faces fines up to 50,000 euros ($61,000) and possible prison terms for its management.[25]

Consumer Confusion and Loss of Benefits

Finally, mandatory GM labeling results in confusion and lost benefits for consumers. For example, GM labeling can impose "cognitive costs" on some consumers, including diluting their attention to more important warnings on food labels and contributing to overwarning that undermines the effectiveness of all consumer warnings.[26] Product warning experts frequently note the importance of limiting and prioritizing information provided by labels regarding health risks of products to promote the effectiveness of such warnings.[27] Mandatory GM labeling contributes to the growing social problem of overwhelming consumers with too much information on food and other product labels, to the extent that many start ignoring all labels, even those containing important information that they really should heed.[28]

Mandatory GM labels also have the potential to affirmatively mislead the public. The American Medical Association, in its 2000 position statement opposing mandatory labeling of GM foods, warned of this possibility:

> Labeling may be misleading not only because of what it says but also because of what it fails to say. With voluntary labeling even truthful information could mislead consumers. For example, does touting a food as not being "genetically modified" imply that there is a danger or defect inherent in products that are

derived from recombinant DNA sources? Such misleading implications must be avoided and the information presented must
appear in its proper context.[29]

The presence of a government-required label would likely be construed by
much of the public as conveying a safety warning of hazard or other important difference associated with GM foods, even though no such hazard or
difference is known to exist.[30] As then secretary of the U.S. Department of
Health and Human Services Tommy Thompson stated in a 2002 speech,
"Mandatory labeling will only frighten consumers. Labeling implies that
biotechnology products are unsafe."[31]

GM food fears are real for many consumers, and governments exacer-
bate and help legitimize them through stigmatizing GM labels.[32] Numerous
studies have found consumer confusion arising from the public's misunder-
standing of terms such as "genetically modified" required on mandatory
labels.[33] The Canadian government undertook a series of focus groups with
consumers to determine how the public would perceive labels stating that a
product contained "genetically modified" ingredients. Some interpreted the
label to mean that chemicals had been added to the food, while others
thought it meant that the crops had not been grown in soil.[34] Indeed, other
surveys have shown that, when asked, most consumers concede they do not
know enough to understand the meaning of a GM label and would need to
be educated before the label could be effective.[35] This potential to mislead
and confuse consumers imposes social costs that make sense only if they are
offset by substantial benefits from labeling GM foods, which previous chapters have demonstrated are minimal if not nonexistent. Moreover, most, if
not all, of the costs, burdens, disruptions, and confusion associated with a
mandatory GM labeling scheme could be avoided with a voluntary labeling
approach, discussed next.

8

A Voluntary Labeling Alternative

Many of the problems with a mandatory GM labeling requirement could be addressed with a voluntary scheme for labeling non-GM products, while giving consumers a true choice of purchasing GM products or not. Any consumer "right to know" could be much better achieved by allowing the segment of the population that wants to avoid GM foods to pay to do so through voluntary labeling.[1] Already consumers have the choice not to buy GM products by buying foods certified as organic. The organic food industry is a rapidly growing segment of the food market, with sales numbers well in excess of those for GM foods.

A voluntary "non-GM" labeling scheme would give consumers an additional option for avoiding GM foods. Specifically, if a company determined that there was a viable consumer demand for products without GM ingredients, it could avoid such inputs and label its products as containing "no GM." Survey data suggest that a non-GM label would be perceived as the most adequate and credible GM-related label by the public.[2] Moreover, experimental studies with consumers have found no preference for mandatory GM labeling over a non-GM labeling scheme, a finding that, according to one set of study authors, "provides evidence that the voluntary labeling policy in the USA is the best policy."[3] Another recent study of market processes and the actual response to mandatory and voluntary GM labeling programs in Europe and Canada also found that the voluntary non-GM approach is more likely to provide consumer choice than mandatory GM labeling.[4]

A market-driven, voluntary labeling approach is both more efficient and fairer to all consumers than mandatory labeling.[5] From an efficiency perspective, if the number of consumers willing to pay extra to have non-GM foods really is significant, then food producers and distributors will have economic incentives to provide such products.[6] There are precedents for such an approach with kosher and halal foods, low-fat foods, and organic foods, whereby it is the consumers seeking such specialized foods who pay any additional costs in ensuring their availability and purity. If actual consumer demand for non-GM foods exists, depending upon the level of purity (that is, the tolerance for GM content), the costs of ensuring such genetic purity of food would decrease with the number of consumers seeking these products; but at very low tolerances, the costs of compliance could be high. As a result, a voluntary label system would allow those consumers to tap into the power of the marketplace to find and pay for such foods without imposing costs on or restricting the choices of others.[7]

From an ethical perspective, a mandatory GM labeling program deprives individual consumers of a personal choice as to whether they wish to pay for such a requirement, since it applies across the board to all products and all consumers. One clear message from the studies on public perception of GM foods is that the population is not homogeneous in their response to them—some consumers oppose GM foods and want to avoid them; some support GM foods and are not concerned about consuming them; and others (perhaps the largest group) are indifferent on the issue.[8] A voluntary non-GM labeling system would fairly and efficiently limit the costs and burdens of the labeling information to those who wish to avoid GM foods and pay the costs of labeling and segregation. As one ethicist has argued,

> It is possible here to distinguish between two types of consumers: those who do not mind buying GM foods (though this group at the time is a minority in most parts of Europe) and those who do not want to buy GM foods. The former group of consumers probably has no clear interest in knowing whether or not a particular product is GMO related, whereas the latter group does have a clear interest in being able to tell whether or not a product is GMO related. Hence, it could be argued that those consumers who have an interest in distinguishing between GM foods and non-GM foods should defray the expenses of labeling; that it, in other words, is the non-GM foods that should be labeled and thereby meet with the extra costs of such a process.[9]

Thus, a non-GM labeling approach has the advantage of not imposing the costs of labeling on those who do find such undertakings to be worth the cost, including many low-income citizens. Studies show that lower-income shoppers are not affected by (and hence do not benefit from) GM labels,[10] yet they would bear a disproportionate burden from the costs of mandatory GM labeling spread across the entire population.

Another advantage of a voluntary scheme is that non-GM suppliers can use a threshold for GM content that is tailored to consumers' level of concern.[11] Such standards can use third-party certifications, analogous to organic certification. Whole Foods Markets recently committed to such a certification process.[12] Such voluntary measures can be tailored to meet the needs, budgets, and any other desire of customers for non-GM products.[13] This approach is adjustable to realities (as Whole Foods may soon learn, given the low 0.9 percent tolerance it is initially endorsing), and a well-managed system may be able to reduce the high costs associated with mandatory GM labeling. One cost surely avoided is that of the increased risk of penalties, including prison sentences in some jurisdictions, that would result from inadvertent, but almost inevitable, noncompliance with arbitrary governmental regulatory tolerances and testing for trace residues.[14]

In January 2001, the FDA issued draft guidelines to assist manufacturers who seek to label their products as "non-GM," or non–genetically engineered. Those guidelines provide that such voluntary labels should not be misleading—for example, a label should not call a food "GM-free" or "not genetically modified," since "free" implies to consumers a zero level that is not feasibly detected or achieved.[15] A recent survey of products in the organic food supermarket Whole Foods found 137 products with non-GM labels, suggesting that a market is developing for such foods for consumers who seek such products.[16] Moreover, a private consortium of food manufacturers, retailers, processors, distributors, farmers, and consumer organizations, the Non-GMO project,[17] has formed to promote and provide certification of foods without GM ingredients, again demonstrating the power of the market to respond to consumer demand. Other nations, including Canada and Germany, have recently adopted standards for voluntary labeling of non-GM foods.[18] Moreover, several EU nations, including France, Germany, Italy, and Austria, have recently adopted voluntary GM-free labeling for products such as meat and eggs produced from livestock fed without GM animal feed, which are exempt from mandatory GM labeling under the existing EU requirement. An additional advantage of a voluntary labeling scheme over a mandatory program is that voluntary standards can be quickly enacted or removed depending on public demand, and adjusted to evolving factual information without the need for lengthy regulatory proceedings.[19]

A voluntary labeling program would also be consistent with the recommendations of the 2002 World Summit on Sustainable Development (WSSD), which endorsed voluntary approaches for satisfying consumers' "right to know" about the processes used in food production. The WSSD adopted the following recommendation to nations:

> Develop and adopt, where appropriate, *on a voluntary basis,* effective, transparent, verifiable, non-misleading and non-discriminatory consumer information tools to provide information relating to sustainable consumption and production, including human health and safety aspects. These tools should not be used as disguised trade barriers.[20]

Finally, unlike a mandatory GM labeling scheme, a voluntary non-GM labeling approach could not be subverted or used to try to banish GM (or any other type of food) from the market. As such, only a voluntary approach will satisfy the often-stated goal of GM proponents and opponents alike of giving consumers a true choice as to whether or not to purchase and consume GM foods.

Conclusion

The case for mandatory labeling of GM foods seems compelling at first glance. Such a requirement would be consistent with apparently overwhelming public support, would promote informed consumer choice in a free market, and would satisfy the consumer's right to know. As the analysis in this book demonstrates, however, none of these rationales stands up to closer scrutiny. While most people support GM labeling in the abstract, they do *not* generally support such a requirement if they are also asked whether they would be willing to pay more for their food to get this information, which would inevitably be the case. Rather than promoting consumer choice, mandatory labeling is used to deprive the public of the choice to purchase GM foods, as the situation in Europe and elsewhere demonstrates. Any alleged "right to know" the GM content of foods would be both infeasible and unfair, likely to mislead and certainly not inform consumers, and inconsistent with the reality and precedent of our food distribution system. Moreover, consumers can avoid GM foods if they so desire by purchasing organic foods or foods voluntarily labeled as non–genetically engineered. In short, the very reasons usually advanced to justify mandatory GM labeling, when investigated more fully, in fact weigh against such a requirement.

GM food labeling not only represents an unsound domestic policy, it also functions as an unwarranted restraint on international trade.[1] The stringent EU traceability and labeling requirements impose an unnecessary and unfair burden on GM food imports from the United States and elsewhere, effectively serving to continue the EU's de facto moratorium on GM products that has already been ruled illegal by the World Trade Organization. The United States and Argentina are particularly well positioned to bring a second WTO complaint against the EU, this time targeting the application of its traceability and labeling requirements to the process of production (for example, for soybean and canola oil that are produced "from" biotech crops).[2]

The GM labeling debate is likely to evolve significantly over the next few years. Biotechnology companies are now working on a second generation of GM foods, including many that are expected to provide enhanced nutritional and other benefits. Foods with these enhanced traits will no longer be "substantially equivalent" to existing foods under the FDA's 1992 policy statement, and therefore may require additional labeling information. Indeed, manufacturers and food processors are likely to seek such labeling voluntarily to capture the premium price associated with such benefits.[3] While the details of such labels have not yet been finalized, it would make sense to require disclosure of the enhanced trait (such as lower fat content or enhanced levels of specific vitamins) rather than the process by which the trait was added (such as genetic modification). As with existing genetically modified crops, it may be possible, at least in some cases, to construct similar changes with other methods, although likely with less precision, and there is no reason to discriminate against genetic engineering.

Finally, mandatory GM labeling is not only a poor public policy decision in its own right, but it would also set a dangerous precedent that would open the floodgates to politically motivated, unscientific labeling requirements. Many of the same activists who push for mandatory GM labels also advocate labeling of irradiated foods, nanotechnology products, and, now, foods from cloned animals (see appendix A). As is the case for GM foods, there is no scientific or health basis for such labeling requirements. Rather, such demands seek to block beneficial new technologies and are not consistent with, or responsible to, the well-being or wishes of the general public.

Appendix A
Animal Cloning: The Latest Skirmish

The latest flurry in the biotechnology labeling controversy is whether meat from cloned animals and their progeny must be labeled. Modern biotechnological techniques have enabled the reproductive cloning of a variety of nonhuman species, some of which are now being commercialized. While much publicity surrounds attempts to market cloned pets,[1] the more serious economic opportunity is the cloning of valuable livestock. Some companies are already beginning preparations to market meat and milk from cloned animals and their progeny, although no such products have been commercialized to date. According to a report in the *Washington Post,* animal cloning "will bring consumers a level of consistency and quality impossible to attain with conventional breeding, making perfectly marbled beef and reliably lean and tasty pork the norm on grocery shelves."[2]

In preparation for receiving applications to market such products, the FDA has conducted a series of activities over the past few years, including a massive risk assessment and a request for public comments. The risk assessment concluded that meat and milk from cloned animals, similar to foods prepared from genetic engineering, appear to present no unique health or environmental risks. The FDA risk assessment found that food derived from clones and their offspring is indistinguishable from that of conventionally reproduced animals.[3] This report was based on hundreds of domestic and international peer-reviewed studies conducted over decades. Several of these studies analyzed multiple generations of animals. The risk assessment followed a report by the National Academy of Sciences that reached a similar conclusion that food products derived from cloned animals do not "present a food safety concern."[4] The EU's European Food Safety Authority reached a similar conclusion, finding that "there is no indication that differences exist in terms of food safety for meat and milk of clones and their progeny compared with those from conventionally bred animals."[5]

The public consultation, in contrast, produced a very different result, with an expression of widespread public concern about the social and ethical aspects of animal cloning. A strongly held sentiment by most of the public commentators was that meat and milk from cloned animals and their progeny should be labeled. In addition, public opinion polling by the Consumers Union found that an "overwhelming majority" of surveyed Americans agreed that milk and meat from cloned animals should be labeled via government mandates.[6] As with GM foods, the basis for such labeling would not be any scientifically established risk, but rather a consumer's right to know. The FDA, applying the longstanding principles and legal precedents discussed in chapter 2, rejected the calls for mandatory labeling of such products based on available scientific evidence.[7]

The FDA's decision has provoked action by some federal and state legislators. Some members of Congress have introduced bills requiring labeling of products from cloned animals, but those bills have not advanced to congressional votes (at least, not as of yet).[8] State laws are likely to be the first movers in regulating labeling of clones. California's SB 63 would have required that meat or milk from animal clones or their progeny be labeled as cloned. Mainstream farm groups opposed this bill,[9] with organic industry advocates and many public interest groups supporting labeling. After its narrow passage through a divided senate (twenty-one to eighteen), Governor Arnold Schwarzenegger vetoed the bill, issuing a press release stating that he did not agree with mandatory labeling.

In the absence of any mandated cloning labeling, the market is already showing signs of responding to consumer concerns, just as has been proposed for GM foods. The meat industry has its own incentives to serve any segment of the United States and worldwide market that shuns any such "clone meat," and the two largest companies producing cloned cattle have recently announced they will create a registry of all cloned animals that can be used to verify clone-free labels.[10] The Biotechnology Industry Organization (BIO) has supported voluntary traceability of cloned meat nationwide.[11] Moreover, while the FDA may approve the sale of cloned foods sometime soon, the livestock breeding industry yielded in 2008 to a request from the U.S. Department of Agriculture for a moratorium until further review of the economic impacts on commercial markets for meat from clones and their offspring could be conducted. Voluntary labeling once again would provide the consumers with choice, while a stigmatizing government-imposed mandatory label would deny them that choice.

Appendix B
National GM Labeling Laws and Policies

Type of GM labeling	Countries that enforce labeling policies	Countries with partially enforced or unenforced labeling policies	Countries with probable plans to introduce a labeling policy
Mandatory	Australia, Brazil, China, European Union, Japan, New Zealand, Norway, Russia, Saudi Arabia, South Korea, Switzerland, Taiwan	Croatia, Ecuador, El Salvador, Indonesia, Malaysia, Mauritius, Serbia, Sri Lanka, Thailand, Ukraine, Vietnam	Nigeria, Uganda, UAE, Zambia
Voluntary	Argentina, Canada, Chile, Hong Kong, Kenya, Philippines, South Africa, USA		Peru

Sources: Adapted from U.S. Department of Agriculture (USDA) GAIN reports (2006–9), http://gain.fas.usda.gov/Pages/Default.aspx (accessed December 16, 2009); G. P. Gruère and S. R. Rao, "A Review of International Labeling Policies of Genetically Modified Food to Evaluate India's Proposed Rule," *AgBioForum* 10 (2007): 51–64; G. P. Gruère and D. Sengupta, "Biosafety at the Crossroads: An Analysis of South Africa's Market and Trade Policies for Genetically Modified Products," IFPRI Discussion Paper 796, 2008, http://www.ifpri.org/publication/biosafety-crossroads (accessed September 15, 2009).

Notes

Introduction

1. See Institute for Responsible Technology, "Petition to President Obama to Support Mandatory Labeling of GM Foods," http://www.responsibletechnology.org/GMFree/TakeAction/MandatoryLabelingPetitiontoObama/index.cfm (accessed September 9, 2009). The same Web page has a "Free Non-GMO Shopping Guide," which presumably satisfies most consumers' "right to know" through voluntary non-GM and organic labels.

2. The United Kingdom–based "Soil Association" and the U.S.–based Organic Consumers Association both cite a "possible" pledge by Obama to support GM labeling. S. Hills, "US Election Impact on GM Food," *Meatprocess,* October 31, 2008, http://www.meatprocess.com/Industry-markets/US-election-impact-on-GM-food (accessed December 14, 2009). There was, however, no indication of that alleged promise on the Obama-Biden campaign website or in any official document or mainstream news report. Moreover, Obama responded in the negative to a direct question posed to him in Iowa regarding GM food labeling in January 2008, and more recently stated in September 2008 (at Science Debate 2008) that "advances in the genetic engineering of plants have provided enormous benefits to American farmers. I believe that we can continue to modify plants safely with new genetic methods," causing anti-biotech activists to declare him "uninformed about GE food" or "choosing to propagate the biotech façade due to industry influence." B. Harrison, "GE Food and the New Administration: Change or More of the Same?" *GM Watch,* December 2008, http://www.organicconsumers.org/articles/article_15866.cfm (accessed December 14, 2009).

3. J. Forster, "GM Foods: Why Fight Labeling?" *Business Week,* November 11, 2002, 44.

4. See, generally, J. Entine (ed.), *Let Them Eat Precaution: How Politics Is Undermining the Genetic Revolution in Agriculture* (Washington, D.C.: AEI Press, 2006).

Chapter 1: Background on GM Foods

1. S. K. Harlander, "The Evolution of Modern Agriculture and Its Future with Biotechnology," *Journal of the American College of Nutrition* 21 (2002): 161S–165S. "Mutagenesis" uses radiation or chemicals to shuffle the genes of an organism into new positions, potentially creating useful new crops (such as herbicide-resistant canola).

2. G. Conko, "Eat, Drink, and Be Merry: Why Mandatory Biotech Food Labeling Is Unnecessary," Cascade Policy Institute, October 2002.

3. A. McHughen, *Pandora's Picnic Basket: The Potential and Hazards of Genetically Modified Foods* (Oxford: Oxford University Press, 2000); Harlander, "The Evolution of Modern Agriculture."

4. National Academy of Sciences, *Introduction of Recombinant DNA-Engineered Organisms into the Environment: Key Issues* (Washington, D.C.: National Academy Press, 1987), 11.

5. C. S. Prakash, "The Genetically Modified Crop Debate in the Context of Agricultural Evolution," *Plant Physiology* 126: 8–15.

6. International Service for the Acquisition of Agri-biotech Applications (ISAAA), "Global Status of Commercialized Biotech/GM Crops: 2008," ISAAA Brief 39-2008: Executive Summary, 2008, http://www.isaaa.org/resources/publications/briefs/39/executivesummary/default.html (accessed September 15, 2009).

7. U.S. Department of Agriculture, Economic Research Service, *Adoption of Genetically Engineered Crops in the U.S.,* July 1, 2009, http://www.ers.usda.gov/data/biotechcrops/ (accessed December 14, 2009).

8. See, for example, U.S. Department of Agriculture, Economic Research Service, *The First Decade of Genetically Engineered Crops in the United States,* Economic Information Bulletin No. 11, April 2006, http://www.ers.usda.gov/publications/eib11/eib11.pdf (accessed September 15, 2009).

9. G. Brookes and P. Barfoot, "Global Impact of Biotech Crops: Socio-Economic and Environmental Effects in the First Ten Years of Commercial Use," *AgbioForum* 9 (2006): 139–51.

10. X. Ye, S. Al-Babili, A. Klöti, J. Zhang, P. Lucca, P. Beyer, and I. Potrykus, "Engineering the Provitamin A (Beta-Carotene) Biosynthetic Pathway into (Carotenoid-Free) Rice Endosperm," *Science* 287, no. 5451 (2000): 303–5. Peter Beyer and Ingo Potrykus developed "Golden Rice" by adding the gene for beta-carotene, a precursor of vitamin A, to rice using genetic engineering. Since no rice cultivars naturally produce this precursor, only GM technologies could be used to accomplish the task. Despite a willingness to donate Golden Rice to developing countries to improve the nutrition and health of their populations, the research team developing it is "working out legal issues," including obstacles posed by GM food labeling laws in many Asian markets. "Golden Rice," *Your World: Biotechnology and You* 1, no. 10 (2000): 10, http://biotech2.newcitymedia. com/resources/pdf/yw10_1.pdf (accessed September 9, 2009). K. R. Curtis, J. J. McCluskey, and T. I. Wahl, "Consumer Acceptance of Genetically Modified Food Products in the Developing World," *AgBioForum* 7 (2004): 70–75 (describing Chinese consumer interest in vitamin-enriched rice, but also demanding labeling of GM content).

11. T. S. Mor, H. S. Mason, D. D. Kirk, C. J. Arntzen, and G. A. Cardineau, "Plants as a Production and Delivery Vehicle for Orally Delivered Subunit Vaccines," in *New Generation Vaccines,* ed. M. M. Levine, G. C. Woodrow, J. B. Kaper, and G. S. Cobon, 3d ed. (New York: Marcel Dekker, 2004).

12. For example, Syngenta announced in mid-2008 that its R&D pipeline included "second generation trait launches" for 2009 onwards, including MIR162 (VIP/broad lep) for broad Lepidoptera insect control; corn amylase for more efficient bioethanol production; and drought-tolerant corn. See Syngenta, "Syngenta Half Year Results 2008: Strong Performance, Positive Outlook," press release, July 24, 2008, www.syngenta.com/en/media/pdf/mediareleases/en/20080724_halfyear_short_en.pdf (accessed September 9, 2009).

13. For a listing of over 230 published studies, see David Tribe, "200+ Published Safety Assessments on GM Foods and Feeds," *GMO Pundit Blog,* June 13, 2007, http://gmopundit.blogspot.com/2007/06/150-published-safety-assessments-on-gm.html (accessed September 9, 2009).

14. See Truth about Trade and Technology, "Counting Up," 2008, http://www. truthabouttrade.org (accessed September 9, 2009).

15. See Joint Research Centre (EU), *Scientific and Technical Contribution to the Development of an Overall Health Strategy in the Area of GMOs: Executive Summary,* 2007, 6, http://ec.europa.eu/dgs/jrc/downloads/jrc_20080910_gmo_study_en.pdf (accessed

September 15, 2009; "No demonstration of any health effect of GM food products submitted to the regulatory process has been reported so far").

16. Quoted in "Access Issues May Determine Whether Agri-Biotech Will Help the World's Poor," *Nature* 402 (1999): 342.

17. See N. Kalaitzandonakes, J. M. Alston, and K. J. Bradford, "Compliance Costs for Regulatory Approval of New Biotech Crops," *Nature Biotechnology* 25 (2007): 509–11.

18. U.S. Food and Drug Administration, "Statement of Policy: Foods Derived from New Plant Varieties," *Federal Register* 57 (May 29, 1992): 22984–23005.

19. National Research Council (NRC), *Genetically Modified Pest-Protected Plants: Science and Regulation* (Washington, D.C.: National Academy Press, 2000), 43.

20. National Research Council, *Environmental Effects of Transgenic Plants* (Washington, D.C.: National Academy Press, 2002), 49.

21. Food and Agriculture Organization/World Health Organization, "Joint FAO/WHO Expert Consultation on Biotechnology and Food Safety," 1996, 4, ftp://ftp.fao.org/es/esn/food/biotechnology.pdf (accessed December 14, 2009).

22. World Health Organization, "20 Questions on Genetically Modified Foods," http://www.who.int/foodsafety/publications/biotech/20questions/en, 3 (accessed September 9, 2009).

23. Food and Agriculture Organization. "The State of Food and Agriculture 2003–2004: Agricultural Biotechnology, Meeting the Needs of the Poor?" 2004, 58, http://www.fao.org/docrep/006/Y5160E/Y5160E00.HTM (accessed December 14, 2009; citations omitted).

24. European Commission, "GMOs: Are There Any Risks?" press release, October 8, 2001, http://ec.europa.eu/research/press/2001/pr0810en.html (accessed September 9, 2009).

Chapter 2: GM Labeling Laws and Regulations

1. Office of Science and Technology Policy, "Coordinated Framework for Regulation of Biotechnology," *Federal Register* 51 (June 26, 1986): 23302–50.

2. U.S. Food and Drug Administration, "Statement of Policy: Foods Derived from New Plant Varieties," *Federal Register* 57 (May 29, 1992): 22984–23005.

3. Organisation of Economic Co-operation and Development (OECD), "Safety Evaluation of Foods Derived by Modern Biotechnology: Concepts and Principles," 1993, 14, http://www.oecd.org/dataoecd/37/18/41036698.pdf (accessed December 14, 2009).

4. U.S. Food and Drug Administration, "Statement of Policy."

5. F. H. Degnan, "Biotechnology and the Food Label," in *Labeling Genetically Modified Food: The Philosophical and Legal Debate,* ed. P. Weirich (Oxford: Oxford University Press, 2007), 23–24.

6. U.S. Food and Drug Administration, "Statement of Policy," 2291.

7. Ibid.

8. *Alliance for Bio-Integrity* v. *Shalala,* 116 F. Supp. 2d 166 (D.D.C. 2000).

9. Ibid., 178–79, quoting *Stauber* v. *Shalala,* 895 F. Supp. 1178, 1193 (W.D. Wis. 1995).

10. See Institute for Responsible Technology, "Non-GMO Shopping Guide," http://www.nongmoshoppingguide.com/SG/Home/index.cfm (accessed December 14, 2009); the Organic Consumers Association, "Why Are GM Foods Not Labeled?" March 2008, http://www.organicconsumers.org/articles/article_17240.cfm (accessed October 27, 2009).

11. U.S. House of Representatives, *Genetically Engineered Food Right to Know Act,* H.R. 5269, 109th Cong. 2d sess. (May 2, 2006).

12. D. Grobe and C. Raab, "Voters' Response to Labeling Genetically Engineered Foods: Oregon's Experience," *Journal of Consumer Affairs* 38 (2004): 320–31.

13. See Organic Consumers Association, "Why Are GM Foods Not Labeled?"

14. European Union Commission Directive 97/35/EC (labeling).

15. Commission Regulation 1829/2003 of the European Parliament and of the Council of 22 September 2003 on genetically modified food and feed: OJ L 268/1, 18.10.2003; Commission Regulation 1830/2003 Concerning the Traceability and Labeling of Genetically Modified Organisms and the Traceability of Food and Feed Products Produced from Genetically Modified Organisms and Amending Directive 2001/18/EC, 2003 O.J. (L 268) 1, recital 11 (September 22, 2003).

16. U.S. Department of Agriculture, Advisory Committee on Biotechnology and 21st Century Agriculture, *Global Traceability and Labeling Requirements for Agricultural Biotechnology Derived Products: Impacts and Implications for the United States,* February 8, 2005, http://www.usda.gov/documents/tlpaperv37final.pdf (accessed September 9, 2009; noting that "the greater the potential for pass-back of various liability claims back up the food and feed chain, the greater the potential impacts on costs and on the sustainability of production and delivery systems").

17. Commission Regulation 1830/2003.

18. Greenpeace Europe, "1 Million Europeans Call for GMO Labelling on Milk, Meat and Eggs," press release, February 5, 2007, http://www.greenpeace.org/eu-unit/press-centre/press-releases2/one-million-petition (accessed September 9, 2009).

19. *Norden,* "Tighter Labelling of GMO Products and GMO-Free Zones in the Nordic Region," October 29, 2008, http://www.norden.org/en/news-and-events/ news/tighter-labelling-of-gmo-products-and-gmo-free-zones-in-the-nordic-region (accessed December 14, 2009).

20. G. P. Gruère and S. R. Rao, "A Review of International Labeling Policies of Genetically Modified Food to Evaluate India's Proposed Rule," *AgBioForum* 10 (2007): 51–64.

21. See Wilna Jansen v Rijssen, "GM Food to be Labelled in South Africa," *Science in Africa,* April 2004, http://www.scienceinafrica.co.za/2004/april/gmlabel.htm (accessed September 9, 2009; discussing proposed labeling of GM in South Africa and noting that "the stricter regulations will come with a price tag of their own—up to 10% increase in the price of GM foods to cover the necessary laboratory tests, tracing and monitoring by government"); Heike Baumüller, *Domestic Import Regulations for Genetically Modified Organisms and Their Compatibility with WTO Rules: Some Key Issues,* Trade Knowledge Network, August 2003, http://www.tradeknowledge network.net/pdf/tkn_domestic_regs.pdf (accessed September 9, 2009).

22. For example, China has not issued regulations stating the tolerance it would permit for GM food, making the presumptive tolerance "zero" in the absence of further guidance.

23. See Gruère and Rao, "A Review of International Labeling Policies."

24. Ibid. See also GeneWatch, "A Short History of GM Labelling: Global Status of GM Labelling Legislation," http://www.genewatch.org/uploads/f03c6d66a9b354535 738483c1c3d49e4/A_Short_History_of_Labelling.pdf (accessed September 10, 2009; erroneously records South Africa as a mandatory GM food labeling nation). Compare G. P. Gruère and D. Sengupta, "Biosafety at the Crossroads: An Analysis of South Africa's Market and Trade Policies for Genetically Modified Products," IFPRI Discussion Paper 796, 2008, http://www.ifpri.org/publication/biosafety-crossroads (accessed September 15, 2009).

25. See K. Ramessar, T. Capell, R. M.Twyman, H. Quemada, and P. Christou, "Trace and Traceability—A Call for Regulatory Harmony," *Nature Biotechnology* 26 (2008): 975–77; Gruère and Rao, "A Review of International Labeling Policies"; Food Standards Australia New Zealand, *Report on the Review of Labelling of Genetically Modified Foods,* December 2003, 2 http://www.foodstandards.gov.au/_src files/GM_label_REVIEW%20REPORT%20_Final%203_.pdf, (accessed December 14, 2009) ("The analysis of international regulations for the labelling of GM foods illustrates that specific food labelling requirements vary markedly from country to

country"); M. F. Teisl and J. A. Caswell, "Information Policy and Genetically Modified Food: Weighing the Benefits and Costs," University of Massachusetts Amherst Department of Resource Economics Working Paper No. 2003-1, 2003, http://courses.umass.edu/resec/workingpapers/documents/resecworkingpaper2003-1.pdf (accessed September 10, 2009).

26. Rameessar et al., "Trace and Traceability"; M. Klintman, "The Genetically Modified (GM) Food Labelling Controversy: Ideological and Epistemic Crossovers," *Social Studies of Science* 32 (2002): 71–91.

27. G. P. Gruère and M. W. Rosegrant, "What Information Should be Required on Shipments of LMO-FFPS? Analyzing Options Under Article 18.2.a of the Biosafety Protocol," PBS Policy Brief 8, 2007, http://www.cbd.int/doc/external/mop-04/ifpri-pbs-policy-08-en.pdf (accessed January 21, 2010).

28. Cartagena Protocol on Biosafety to the Convention on Biological Diversity, 2000, http://www.cbd.int/biosafety.

29. During Free Trade Agreement talks with the United States, Malaysia environment minister Azmi Khalid said Malaysia's position on GM food labeling would be "consistent with that of Australia and the European Union," and that proposed legislation on biosafety was expected to be passed by parliament and come into force by late 2007, with GM labeling made mandatory soon after that. See Malaysia's Biosafety Act 2007 (Act 678), http://www.nre.gov.my/EN/Pages/BioSafety.aspx (accessed September 14, 2009) or through the Biosafety Clearing House portal, http://bch.cbd.int. See also NRE Malaysia, with Centre of Excellence for Biodiversity Law (CEBLAW) law faculty, *The Biosafety Act of Malaysia: Dispelling the Myths,* October 28, 2008, http://www.nre.gov.my/EN/Publication/FAQFinalFinal.pdf (accessed September 15, 2009); S. M. Mohamed Idris, "Biosafety Bill: Sound Reasons for the Label," *Political Friendster* blog, May 30, 2007, http://www.politicalfriendster.com/showConnection.php?id1=3151&id2=5433 (accessed September 14, 2009).

30. See G. P. Gruère and N. W. Rosegrant, "Assessing the Implementation Effects of the Biosafety Protocol's Proposed Stringent Information Requirements for Genetically Modified Commodities in Countries of the Asia Pacific Economic Cooperation," *Review of Agricultural Economics* 30: 214–32.

31. World Trade Organization, "European Communities: Measures Affecting the Approval and Marketing of Biotech Products," WT/DS291/R, WT/DS292/R, WT/DS293/R, 2006, http://www.wto.org/english/tratop_e/dispu_e/cases_e/ds291_e.htm (accessed December 14, 2009).

32. P. Brown, "US Threatens WTO Reprisals over EU Labels on GE Food," *Guardian* (London), July 31, 2000, http://www.organicconsumers.org/ge/USvsWTO.cfm (accessed September 14, 2009).

33. S. Charnovitz, "The Supervision of Health and Biosafety Regulation by World Trade Rules," *Tulane Environmental Law Journal* 13 (2000): 271–302.

34. World Trade Organization, "Report of the Appellate Body: EC Hormones Concerning Meat and Meat Products (Hormones)," WT/DS26/AB/R, WT/DS48/AB/R, AB-1997-4, January 16, 1998. See also T. P. Stewart and D. S. Johanson, "The WTO Beef Hormone Dispute: An Analysis of the Appellate Body Decision," *U.C. Davis Journal of International Law and Policy* 5 (1999): 219–57; I. Cheyne, "Gateways to the Precautionary Principle in WTO Law," *Journal of Environmental Law* 19 (2007): 155–72.

35. See N. Huei-Chih, "Can Article 5.7 of the WTO SPS Agreement be a Model for the Precautionary Principle?" http://www.law.ed.ac.uk/ahrc/script-ed/vol4-4/huei-chih.asp (accessed October 27, 2009).

36. S. Zarrilli, *International Trade in GMOs and GM Products: National and Multilateral Legal Frameworks,* United Nations Conference on Trade and Development, UNCTAD/ITCD/TAB/30, 2005, 43, http://www.unctad.org/en/docs/itcd tab30_en.pdf (accessed September 14, 2009).

37. See M. Mansour and S. Key, "From Farm to Fork: The Impact on Global Commerce of the New European Union Biotechnology Regulatory Scheme," *International Lawyer* 38 (2004): 55–70.

Chapter 3: The "Right to Know"

1. T. O. McGarity, "Seeds of Distrust: Federal Regulation of Genetically Modified Foods," *University of Michigan Journal of Law Reform* 35 (2002): 403–510.

2. K. Hansen, "Does Autonomy Count in Favor of Labeling Genetically Modified Food?" *Journal of Agricultural and Environmental Ethics* 17 (2004): 67–76.

3. U.S. Food and Drug Administration, "Statement of Policy."

4. J. H. Beales, "Modification and Consumer Information: Modern Biotechnology and the Regulation of Information," *Food and Drug Law Journal* 55 (2000): 105–17.

5. J. Hodgson, "European Parliament Vote Encourages Industry to Proclaim Green Biotech," *Nature Biotechnology* 20 (2002): 756–57 (quoting then EU commissioner for health and consumer affairs David Byrne).

6. P. H. Sand, "Labeling Genetically Modified Food: The Right to Know," *Review of European Community and International Environmental Law* 15 (2006): 185; H. Siipi, and

S. Uusitalo, "Consumer Autonomy and Sufficiency of GMF Labeling," *Journal of Agricultural and Environmental Ethics* 21 (2008): 353–69; A. Rubel and R. Streiffer, "Respecting the Autonomy of European and American Consumers: Defending Positive Labels on GM Foods," *Journal of Agricultural and Environmental Ethics* 18 (2005): 75–84.

7. Hodgson, "European Parliament Vote Encourages Industry."

8. U.S. House of Representatives, *Genetically Engineered Food Right to Know Act,* H.R. 5269, 109th Cong., 2d sess. (May 2, 2006), ·2(5).

9. M. Klintman, "The Genetically Modified (GM) Food Labelling Controversy: Ideological and Epistemic Crossovers," *Social Studies of Science* 32 (2002): 71–91.

10. Rubel and Streiffer, "Respecting the Autonomy of European and American Consumers."

11. Nuffeld Council on Bioethics, *Genetically Modified Crops: The Ethical and Social Issues,* 1999, http://www.nuffieldbioethics.org/fileLibrary/pdf/gmcrop.pdf (accessed September 14, 2009).

12. A. McHughen, "Uninformation and the Choice Paradox," *Nature Biotechnology* 18 (2000): 1018–19.

13. M. F. Teisl, L. Garner, B. Roe, M. E. Vayda, "Labeling Genetically Modified Foods: How Do US Consumers Want to See It Done?" *AgBioForum* 6 (2003): 48–54; Siipi and Uusitalo, "Consumer Autonomy and Sufficiency."

14. McHughen, "Uninformation and the Choice Paradox."

15. Ibid.

16. N. Kalaitzandonakes, "Another Look at Biotech Regulation," *Regulation,* Spring 2004, 44–50; P. Callahan and S. Kilman, "Seeds of Doubt: Some Ingredients Are Genetically Modified Despite Labels' Claims," *Wall Street Journal,* April 5, 2001, A1.

17. A. Pollack, A., "Labeling Genetically Altered Food Is Thorny Issue," *New York Times,* September 26, 2000.

18. McHughen, "Uninformation and the Choice Paradox."

19. Kalaitzandonakes, "Another Look at Biotech Regulation."

20. P. Markie, "Mandatory Genetic Engineering Labels and Consumer Autonomy," in *Labeling Genetically Modified Food: The Philosophical and Legal Debate,* ed. P. Weirich, 88–105 (Oxford: Oxford University Press, 2007).

21. Ibid.; Beales, "Modification and Consumer Information."

22. Center for Science in the Public Interest (CSPI), "National Opinion Poll on Labeling of Genetically Modified Foods," Conducted by Bruskin Research, March 30–April 1, 2001, http://www.cspinet.org/new/poll_gefoods.html (accessed September 14, 2009).

23. K. A. Goldman, "Labeling of Genetically Modified Foods: Legal and Scientific Issues," *Georgetown International Environmental Law Review* 12 (2000): 717–60.

24. *Int'l Dairy Foods Ass'n* v. *Amestoy,* 92 F.3d 67 (2d Cir. 1996), 74. See also *Stauber* v. *Shalala,* 895 F.Supp. 1178 (W.D. Wisc. 1995) ("It is doubtful whether the FDA would even have the power under the [Food, Drug, and Cosmetic Act] to require labeling in a situation where the sole justification for such a requirement is consumer demand").

25. *Alliance for Bio-Integrity* v. *Shalala,* 116 F. Supp. 2d 166 (D.D.C. 2000).

26. Hansen, "Does Autonomy Count?"

Chapter 4: Consumer Choice

1. Greenpeace International, "Policy Concerning the Labelling and Declaration of Genetically Engineered Food Products," November 1997, http://archive.greenpeace.org/comms/97/geneng/policy.html (accessed December 15, 2009).

2. BEUC, the European Consumers' Organisation, "Genetically Modified Foods Campaign for Consumer Choice: New Revised Policy Position," http://www.beuc.eu/BEUCNoFrame/Docs/5/DKJEHKFDBAOFILMKDFBEPEJKPDBY9DBW2Y9DW3571KM/BEUC/docs/DLS/2002-00851-01-E.pdf (accessed December 15, 2009).

3. American Public Health Association, "Support of the Labeling of Genetically Modified Foods," *American Journal of Public Health* 92 (2002): 463.

4. G. P. Gruère, "A Preliminary Comparison of the Retail Level Effects of Genetically Modified Food Labelling Policies in Canada and France," *Food Policy* 31 (2006): 148–61.

5. Ibid.

6. M. Townshead, "Supermarkets Tell Blair: We Won't Stock GM," *Observer* (London), June 8, 2003; N. Kalaitzandonakes and J. Bijman, "Who is Driving Biotechnology Acceptance?" *Nature Biotechnology* 21 (2003): 366–69.

7. G. P. Gruère and S. R. Rao, "A Review of International Labeling Policies of Genetically Modified Food to Evaluate India's Proposed Rule," *AgBioForum* 10 (2007): 51–64.

8. S. Miller, "EU's New Rules Will Shake Up Market for Bioengineered Food," *Wall Street Journal,* April 16, 2004, A1; Greenpeace, "100 Days of GMO Labelling; Consumer Rejection Holds," press release, Brussels/Berlin, July 26, 2004.

9. Gruère, "A Preliminary Comparison of the Retail Level Effects."

10. Ibid.

11. Ibid.

12. Ibid.

13. Greenpeace International, "Policy Concerning the Labelling and Declaration."

14. M. Klintman, "The Genetically Modified (GM) Food Labelling Controversy: Ideological and Epistemic Crossovers," *Social Studies of Science* 32 (2002): 91n61.

15. EAT2K, "Labeling Biotechnology and the Organic Lobby," January 25, 2000, http://archives.foodsafety.ksu.edu/agnet/2000/1-2000/ag-01-31-00-02.txt (accessed September 14, 2009).

16. C. A. Carter and G. P. Gruère, "Mandatory Labeling of Genetically Modified Foods: Does It Really Provide Consumer Choice?" *AgBioForum* 6 (2003): 69.

17. Kalaitzandonakes and Bijman, "Who Is Driving Biotechnology Acceptance?"

18. Center for Science in the Public Interest (CSPI), "National Opinion Poll on Labeling of Genetically Modified Foods."

19. Miller, "EU's New Rules Will Shake Up Market."

20. Carter and Gruère, "Mandatory Labeling of Genetically Modified Foods."

21. Klintman, "The Genetically Modified (GM) Food Labelling Controversy."

22. United Nations Development Programme, *Human Development Report 2001: Making New Technologies Work for Human Development* (New York, N.Y.: Oxford University Press, 2001), 2.

23. Ibid., 3.

24. Ibid.

Chapter 5: Public Opinion

1. Consumers Union, "Why We Need Labeling of Genetically Engineered Food," April 1998, http://www.consumersunion.org/food/whywenny798.htm (accessed September 14, 2009).

2. A. Rubel and R. Streiffer, "Respecting the Autonomy of European and American Consumers: Defending Positive Labels on GM Foods," *Journal of Agricultural and Environmental Ethics* 18 (2005): 75–84.

3. Center for Food Safety, "Summary of U.S. Consumer Polls on GE Foods," http://www.organicconsumers.org/ge/gepolls.cfm (accessed December 15, 2009; listing poll results from numerous organizations).

4. Center for Food Policy, "New National Poll: 88% of US Consumers Want Labels on Genetically Engineered Food," 2002, http://www.foodsafetynow.org/page201.cfm (accessed December 15, 2009).

5. W. K. Hallman, W. C. Hebden, C. L. Cuite, H. L. Aquino, and J. T. Lang, *Americans and GM Food: Knowledge, Opinion and Interest in 2004,* publication number RR-1104-007, Food Policy Institute, Cook College, Rutgers University, 2004, http://www.foodpolicyinstitute.org/docs/pubs/2004_Americans%20and%20GM%20Food_Knowledge%20Opinion%20&%20Interest%20in%202004.pdf (accessed September 15, 2009).

6. International Food Information Council, *Food Biotechnology: A Study of U.S. Consumer Attitudinal Trends* (October 2008), http://www.ific.org/research/biotechres.cfm (accessed October 28, 2009).

7. Center for Science in the Public Interest (CSPI), "National Opinion Poll on Labeling of Genetically Modified Foods," Conducted by Bruskin Research, March 30–April 1, 2001, http://www.cspinet.org/new/poll_gefoods.html (accessed September 14, 2009).

8. International Food Information Council, *Food Biotechnology.*

9. A. Rimal, W. Moon, and S. K. Balasubramanian, "Labelling Genetically Modified Food Products: Consumers' Concern in the United Kingdom," *International Journal of Consumer Studies* 31 (2007): 436–42.

10. L. A. Heslop, "If We Label It, Will They Care? The Effect of GM-Ingredient Labeling on Consumer Responses," *Journal of Consumer Policy* 29 (2006): 203–28.

11. Ibid.

12. C. Noussair, S. Robin, and B. Ruffieux, "Do Consumers Not Care About Biotech Foods or Do They Just Not Read the Labels?" *Economic Letters* 75 (2002): 47–53.

13. M. M. Wolf, A. Stephens, and N. Pedrazzi, "Using Simulated Test Marketing to Examine Purchase Interest in Food Products that are Positioned as GMO-Free," in *Consumer Acceptance of Genetically Modified Food,* ed. R. E. Evenson and V. Santaniello, 53–59 (Cambridge, Mass.: CAB International, 2004).

14. N. Kalaitzandonakes and J. Bijman, "Who is Driving Biotechnology Acceptance?" *Nature Biotechnology* 21 (2003): 366–69; C. Noussair, S. Robin, and B. Ruffieux, "Do Consumers Really Refuse to Buy Genetically Modified Food?" *Economic Journal* 114 (2003): 102–20; N. Kalaitzandonakes, L. A. Marks, and S. S. Vickner, "Consumer Response to Mandated Labeling of Genetically Modified Foods," in *Labeling Genetically Modified Food: The Philosophical and Legal Debate,* ed. P. Weirich, 106–27 (Oxford: Oxford University Press, 2007).

15. L. A. Marks, N. Kalaitzandonakes, and S. S. Vickner, "Consumer Purchasing Behavior towards GM Foods in the Netherlands," in *Consumer Acceptance of Genetically Modified Food,* ed. R. E. Evenson and V. Santaniello, 23–39 (Cambridge, Mass.: CAB International, 2004).

16. F. Zhong, X. Chen, and X. Ye, "GM Food Labeling Policy and Consumer Preference: A Case Study of Actual Edible Oil Sales in Nanjing Supermarkets," *China Economic Quarterly* 5 (2006): 1311–18; X. Chen, F. Zhong, and B. Zhou, "Do Consumers Really Care about Biotech Food Label? What Do We Know? What Else Should We Know?" (paper presented at Southern Agricultural Economics Association Annual Meeting, Atlanta, Ga., January 31–February 3, 2009), http://ideas.repec.org/p/ags/saeana/46198.html (accessed September 15, 2009).

17. Chen et al., "Do Consumers Really Care About Biotech?"

18. European Commission, *Do European Consumers Buy GM Foods? Final Report*, project no. 518435, October 14, 2008, 1-9-1-10, http://www.whybiotech.com/resources/tps/DoConsumersBuyGMFoods.pdf (accessed September 15, 2009).

19. Ibid., 1–11.

20. D. Grobe and C. Raab, "Voters' Response to Labeling Genetically Engineered Foods: Oregon's Experience," *Journal of Consumer Affairs* 38 (2004): 320–31.

21. G. P. Gruère and S. R. Rao, "A Review of International Labeling Policies of Genetically Modified Food to Evaluate India's Proposed Rule," *AgBioForum* 10 (2007): 51–64.

22. M. Reiss, "Labeling GM Foods: The Ethical Way Forward," *Nature Biotechnology* 20 (2002): 868.

23. P. W. B. Phillips and G. Isaac, "GMO Labeling: Threat or Opportunity?" *AgBioForum* 1 (1998): 25–30.

24. K. A. Goldman, "Labeling of Genetically Modified Foods: Legal and Scientific Issues," *Georgetown International Environmental Law Review* 12 (2000): 717–60; W. E. Huffman, "Production, Identity Preservation, and Labeling in a Marketplace with Genetically Modified and Non-genetically Modified Foods," *Plant Physiology* 134 (2004): 3–10; D. S. Bullock and M. Desquilbet, "The Economics of Non-GMO Segregation and Identity Preservation," *Food Policy* 27 (2002): 81–99.

25. Center for Science in the Public Interest (CSPI), "National Opinion Poll on Labeling of Genetically Modified Foods."

26. S. Smyth and P. W. B. Phillips, "Labeling to Manage Marketing of GM Foods," *Trends in Biotechnology* 21 (2003): 389–93.

27. W. Moon and S. K. Balasubramanian, "Willingness to Pay for Non-biotech Foods in the U.S. and the U.K.," *Journal of Consumer Affairs* 37 (2003): 317–39.

28. Ibid., 335.

29. K. Blumenschein, M. Johannesson, G. C. Blomquist, B. Liljas, and R. M. O'Connor, "Experimental Results on Expressed Certainty and Hypothetical Bias in

Contingent Valuation," *Southern Economic Journal* 65 (1998): 169–77; H. Neill, R. G. Cummings, P. Ganderton, G. Harrison, and T. McGuckin, "Hypothetical Surveys and Real Economic Commitments," *Land Economics* 70 (1994): 145–54; Noussair et al., "Do Consumers Really Refuse to Buy?"; Kalaitzandonakes et al., "Consumer Response to Mandated Labeling."

30. M. L. Loureiro and S. Hine, "Preferences and Willingness to Pay for GM Labeling Policies," *Food Policy* 29 (2004): 467–83.

31. Ibid., 479.

32. B. Onyango, R. M. Nayga, and R. Govindasamy, "U.S. Consumers' Willingness to Pay for Food Labeled 'Genetically Modified,'" *Agricultural and Resource Economics Review* 35 (2006): 299–310.

33. W. E. Huffman, J. F. Shogren, M. Rousu, and A. Tegene, "Consumer Willingness to Pay for Genetically Modified Food Labels in a Market with Diverse Information: Evidence from Experimental Auctions," *Journal of Agricultural and Resource Economics* 28 (2003): 481–502.

Chapter 6: Tracking and Surveillance Applications

1. See, for example, E. Conis, "If Genetically Modified Foods Are Out There, Should They Be Labeled as Such? *Los Angeles Times,* October 22, 2007 (quoting Andrew Kimbrell of the Center for Food Safety as stating: "Without labeling, we don't have the ability to prove them [GM foods] unsafe"); J. Bardon, "Scientists Push for GM Labelling," *ABC News (Australia),* October 24, 2008, http://www.abc.net.au/news/stories/2008/10/24/2400428.htm (accessed September 15, 2009).

2. C. Ness, "Food Conscious: The Shopper's GMO Guide," *San Francisco Chronicle,* June 27, 2007.

3. Jason Clay, *World Agriculture and Environment: A Commodity-by-Commodity Guide to Impacts and Practices* (Washington, D.C.: Island Press, 2004), 31.

4. Japan Economic Newswire, "L-Tryptophan Case Costs Showa Denko 205 bil. Yen," August 2, 1996, annex 3, http://www.greenpeace.it/archivio/soia/mialg.htm (accessed September 15, 2009).

5. See United Kingdom, Committee on Toxicity of Chemicals in Food, Consumer Products and the Environment, *COT Statement on L-Tryptophan and Eosinophilia-Myalgia Syndrome,* June 2004, http://www.food.gov.uk/multimedia/pdfs/tryptophan amend200401.pdf (accessed September 15, 2009).

6. U.S. Food and Drug Administration, "Information Paper on L-Tryptophan and 5-Hydroxy-L-Tryptophan, February 2001, http://vm.cfsan.fda.gov/~dms/ds-tryp1. html (accessed September 15, 2009); compare D. W. Manders, "The FDA Ban of L-Tryptophan: Politics, Profits and Prozac," *Social Policy* 26 (2005): 55–58.

7. Reuters, "Woman Wins $1 Million in Showa Denko L-Tryptophan Suit," April 14, 1993, www.greenpeace.it/archivio/soia/mialg.htm (accesed September 15, 2009). Coauthor Thomas Redick was on the defense team for this first trial of a bellwether plaintiff (*Di Rosa v. Showa Denko KK* et al.), in which defendants did not contest medical causation, and no proof of a particular cause was argued or found (that is, the genetic engineering process was *not* established as the cause of harm) in a $1 million damage award. The jury did not award punitive damages, despite plaintiff's request for $110 million.

8. See, for example, Commission Regulation 1829/2003 of the European Parliament and of the Council of 22 September 2003 on genetically modified food and feed: OJ L 268/1, 18.10.2003.

9. J. H. Beales, "Modification and Consumer Information: Modern Biotechnology and the Regulation of Information," *Food and Drug Law Journal* 55 (2000): 105–17.

10. The non-GMO marketplace, which dominates food production in products using corn or soybean ingredients with detectable proteins, might provide researchers with a "control group" of consumers who avoid consumption of genetically modified ingredients. This control group provides a population that has minimized its exposure to genetically modified ingredients, possibly enabling retrospective studies of health effects on the rest of the population where particular corn products (such as snack food and tortillas) are found to contain significant GM corn proteins.

11. S. H. Morris, "EU Biotech Crop Regulations and Environmental Risk: A Case of the Emperor's New Clothes," *Trends in Biotechnology* 25 (2007): 2–6.

12. T. O. McGarity, "Frankenfood Free: Consumer Sovereignty, Federal Regulation, and Industry Control in Marketing and Choosing Food in the United States," in *Labeling Genetically Modified Food: The Philosophical and Legal Debate,* ed. P. Weirich, 128–51 (Oxford: Oxford University Press, 2007); R. S. Greenberger, "Motley Group Pushes for FDA Labels on Biofoods to Help Religious People Observe Dietary Laws," *Wall Street Journal,* August 18, 1999, A20; Siipi and Uusitalo, "Consumer Autonomy."

13. McGarity, "Frankenfood Free."

14. Ibid.

15. H. Miller, "A Rational Approach to Labeling Biotech-Derived Foods," *Science* 284 (1999):1471–72 (citation omitted).

16. Siipi and Usitalo, "Consumer Autonomy and Sufficiency," argue that "even if these kind of foods may not be available at the market yet, they may well be in the future." However, the only examples they identify of products under development that contain genes of potential concern to the dietary practices of some religious groups are, as they concede, medical rather than food products. Ibid., 354 n1.

17. C. L. Richard, "Why Biotech Foods Are Kosher," *O Hebrew,* April 2000, http://www.agbioworld.org/biotech-info/religion/kosher.html (accessed September 15, 2009; noting that the Orthodox Union's Rabbinical Board concluded that "biotech foods do not present Kashruth problems").

18. R. Owen, "Vatican Says GM Food Is a Blessing," *The Times (London),* August 5, 2003, http://www.agbioworld.org/biotech-info/religion/blessing.html (accessed September 15, 2009; stating that the Vatican had declared that GM foods "hold the answer to world starvation and malnutrition").

19. K. Hazzah, "Are GMOs Halal?: Yes, Today's Biotechnology Products Are Approved as Halal," *AgBioView Newsletter,* August 4, 2000, http://www.agbioworld.org/biotech-info/religion/halal.html (accessed September 15, 2009; "according to the Islamic Jurisprudence Council (IJC), foods derived from biotechnology-improved (GMO) crops are halal—fit for consumption by Muslims").

20. *Alliance for Bio-Integrity v. Shalala,* 116 F. Supp. 2d 166, 181 (D.D.C. 2000).

21. M. Reiss, reply to letter to the editor, *Nature Biotechnology* 20 (2002): 1082.

22. American Medical Association (AMA), *Report 10 of the Council on Scientific Affairs: Genetically Modified Crops and Foods,* 2000, http://www.ama-assn.org/ama/no-index/about-ama/13595.shtml (accessed September 15, 2009).

Chapter 7: Costs and Burdens of Mandatory GM Labeling

1. D. S. Bullock and M. Desquilbet, "The Economics of Non-GMO Segregation and Identity Preservation," *Food Policy* 27 (2002): 81–99.

2. R. Weiss, "Food War Claims Its Casualties: High-Tech Crop Fight Victimizes Farmers," *Washington Post,* September 12, 1999, A1.

3. J. A. Caswell, "Labeling Policy for GMOs: To Each His Own?" *Ag BioForum* 3 (2000): 53–57.

4. K. A. Goldman, "Labeling of Genetically Modified Foods: Legal and Scientific Issues," *Georgetown International Environmental Law Review* 12 (2000): 717–60.

5. P. W. B. Phillips and H. Foster, "Labelling for GM Foods: Theory and Practice," (unpublished paper presented at International Consortium on Agricultural Biotechnology Research conference, Ravello, Italy, August 24–28, 2000), abstract available at http://www.economia.uniroma2.it/Conferenze/icabr00/abstracts/philli-fost.htm (accessed September 15, 2009).

6. KPMG Consulting, "Economic Impact Study: Potential Costs of Mandatory Labelling of Food Products Derived from Biotechnology in Canada," Ottawa, December 2000.

7. S. Smyth and P. Phillips, "Competitors Co-operating: Establishing a Supply Chain to Manage Genetically Modified Canola," *International Food and Agribusiness Management Review* 4 (2002): 51–66.

8. W. E. Huffman, J. F. Shogren, M. Rousu, and A. Tegene, "Consumer Willingness to Pay for Genetically Modified Food Labels in a Market with Diverse Information: Evidence from Experimental Auctions," *Journal of Agricultural and Resource Economics* 28 (2003): 481–502.

9. A. McHughen, "Uninformation and the Choice Paradox," *Nature Biotechnology* 18 (2000): 1018–19; KPMG Consulting, "Report on the Costs of Labelling Genetically Modified Foods," Canberra, March 2000; Thomas Bernauer, *Genes, Trade, and Regulation: The Seeds of Conflict in Food Biotechnology* (Princeton, N.J.: Princeton University Press, 2003; GM labels caused significant loss of US export markets to the EU for corn and soybeans).

10. See R. G. Ginder, "GMO Labeling: Effects On Core Business: Objectives in the Grains Value Chain," 1999, http://www.extension.iastate.edu/NR/rdonlyres/DA0B851A-60B8-48FA-8642-0062A76A3EB3/0/gindervc.pdf (accessed September 15, 2009).

11. See G.P. Gruère, C.A. Carter and Y.H. Farzin, "What Labelling Policy for Consumer Choice? The Case of Genetically Modified Food in Canada and Europe," *Canadian Journal of Economics* 41 (2008): 1472–97.

12. American Seed Trade Association, "Seed Purity: Understanding Label Information and Industry Practices," press release, July 12, 2005, http://www.amseed.com/newsDetail.asp?id=118 (accessed September 15, 2009).

13. See, for example, F. Weighardt, "European GMO Labeling Thresholds Impractical and Unscientific," *Nature Biotechnology* 24 (2006): 23–25.

14. R. N. Wisner, "Evolution of the Demand for non-GMO Corn and Soybean," September 15, 1999, www.econ.iastate.edu/faculty/wisner/Wisner/Pages/gmomarci.pdf (accessed September 15 2009).

15. See L. Heller, "Codex and the GM Trade Stalemate," *Food Production Daily.com,* 2007, http://www.foodnavigator-usa.com/Financial-Industry/Codex-and-the-GM-trade-stalemate (accessed December 16, 2009).

16. American Soybean Association, "ASA Calls EU Traceability and Labeling Review a Whitewash," May 10, 2006, press release, http://www.soygrowers.com/newsroom/releases/2006_releases/r051006b.htm (accessed December 16, 2009).

17. EurActiv, "'Crisis looming' as EU blocks GM-Soy imports," October 23, 2009, http://www.euractiv.com/en/cap/crisis-looming-eu-blocks-gm-soy-imports/article-186681 (accessed December 16, 2009).

18. See P. Mitchell, "Europe's Anti-GM Stance to Presage Animal Feed Shortage?" *Nature Biotechnology* 110 (2007): 1065–66.

19. D. S. Doering, *Designing Genes: Aiming for Safety and Sustainability in U.S. Agriculture and Biotechnology* (Washington, D.C.: World Resources Institute, 2004).

20. R. L. Paarlberg, "Technology Adoption in Developing Countries: The Case of Genetically Modified Crops," 2003, http://www.au.af.mil/au/awc/awcgate/cia/nic 2020/technology_adoption_nov6.pdf (accessed September 15, 2009).

21. Japan banned imports of U.S. rice outright after the disclosure of the contamination, while the EU imposed testing requirements for each shipment of U.S. rice that were costly enough effectively to close the market to U.S. rice exports. See *New York Times,* "European Restrictions on Rice Imports," August 24, 2006. The contaminated rice violated not only the EU's and Japan's GM labeling requirements but also their GM authorization regulations, since the Liberty Link strain had never been approved for sale in any country.

22. L. Partos, "Costs to Food Business to Rise If GM Zero-Tolerance Prevails, Warns CIAA," *Food Navigator.com,* June 16, 2008.

23. *Rickmers Reismuehle GMBH* v. *Riceland Foods, Inc.,* U.S. District Court (W.D. AK) Case 4:07-cv-00733-JMM (filed 08/21/2007). See also AP Newswire, "German Company Sues Ark. Rice Millers over Modified Rice," August 23, 2007, www.agbios.com/main.php?action=ShowNewsItem&id=8746 (accessed September 15, 2009).

24. See *In Re Genetically Modified Rice Litigation,* 251 F.R.D. 392 (E.D. Mo. 2009).

25. J. Koester, "Certified Non-GM Ingredients a Must to Avoid GM Labeling in EU," *Non-GMO Report,* October 12, 2005, 13, http://www.non-gm-farmers.com/news_print.asp?ID=2478 (accessed December 16, 2009).

26. M. F. Teisl and J. A. Caswell, "Information Policy and Genetically Modified Food: Weighing the Benefits and Costs," University of Massachusetts Amherst

Working Paper No. 2003-1, 2003, http://courses.umass.edu/resec/workingpapers/ documents/resecworkingpaper2003-1.pdf (accessed September 15, 2009).

27. G. J. S. Wilde, "The Theory of Risk Homeostasis: Implications for Safety and Health," *Risk Analysis* 2 (1982): 209–25.

28. Ibid. See also Teisl and Caswell, "Information Policy and Genetically Modified Food"; T. Parker-Poe, "Danger: Warning Labels May Backfire," *Wall Street Journal,* April 28, 1997, B1.

29. American Medical Association (AMA), *Report 10 of the Council on Scientific Affairs: Genetically Modified Crops and Foods,* 2000, http://www.ama-assn.org/ama/no-index/about-ama/13595.shtml (accessed September 15, 2009).

30. H. I. Miller and P. VanDoren, "Food Risks and Labeling Controversies," *Regulation* 23, no. 1 (2000): 35–39.

31. P. Elias, "White House Opposes Biotech Labels," *Washington Post,* June 10, 2002.

32. See, for example, D. Normile, "Asia Gets a Taste of Genetic Food Fights," *Science* 289 (2000): 1279–81.

33. M. F. Teisl, L. Halverson, K. O'Brien, B. Roe, N. Ross, and M. Vayda, "Focus Group Reactions to Genetically Modified Food Labels," *AgBioForum* 5 (2002): 6–9; W. K. Hallman, W. C. Hebden, C. L. Cuite, H. L. Aquino, and J. T. Lang, *Americans and GM Food: Knowledge, Opinion and Interest in 2004,* publication number RR-1104-007, Food Policy Institute, Cook College, Rutgers University, 2004, http://www.foodpolicy institute.org/docs/pubs/2004_Americans%20and%20GM%20Food_Knowledge %20Opinion%20&%20Interest%20in%202004.pdf (accessed September 15, 2009).

34. M. Potter, "Rhetoric Rules in Altered-Food Debate," *Toronto Star,* March 5, 2000, B1.

35. Teisl et al., "Focus Group Reactions."

Chapter 8: A Voluntary Labeling Alternative

1. N. Kalaitzandonakes, "Another Look at Biotech Regulation," *Regulation,* Spring 2004, 44–50.

2. B. Roe and M. F. Teisl, "Genetically Modified Food Labeling: The Impacts of Message and Messenger on Consumer Perceptions of Labels and Products," *Food Policy* 32 (2007): 49–66.

3. W. E. Huffman, M. Rousu, J. F. Shogren, and A. Tegene, "The Welfare Effects of Implementing Mandatory GM Labeling in the USA," in *Consumer Acceptance of*

Genetically Modified Food, ed. R. E. Evenson and V. Santaniello (Wallingford, U.K.: CAB International, 2004).

4. See G.P. Gruère, C.A. Carter and Y.H. Farzin, "What Labelling Policy for Consumer Choice? The Case of Genetically Modified Food in Canada and Europe," *Canadian Journal of Economics* 41 (2008): 1472–97.

5. M. Reiss, "Labeling GM Foods: The Ethical Way Forward, *Nature Biotechnology* 20 (2002): 868.

6. J. H. Beales, "Modification and Consumer Information: Modern Biotechnology and the Regulation of Information," *Food and Drug Law Journal* 55 (2000): 105–17.

7. M. Mansour and S. Key, "From Farm to Fork: The Impact on Global Commerce of the New European Union Biotechnology Regulatory Scheme," *International Lawyer* 38 (2004): 55–70.

8. M. F. Teisl, S. Radas, and B. Roe, "Struggles in Optimal Labeling: How Different Consumers React to Various Labels for Genetically Modified Foods," *International J. Consumer Studies* 32 (2008): 447–56.

9. K. Hansen, "Does Autonomy Count in Favor of Labeling Genetically Modified Food?" *Journal of Agricultural and Environmental Ethics* 17 (2004): 71.

10. X. Chen, F. Zhong, and B. Zhou, "Do Consumers Really Care about Biotech Food Label? What Do We Know? What Else Should We Know?" (paper presented at Southern Agricultural Economics Association Annual Meeting, Atlanta, Ga., January 31–February 3, 2009), http://ideas.repec.org/p/ags/saeana/46198.html (accessed September 15, 2009).

11. A. McHughen, "Uninformation and the Choice Paradox," *Nature Biotechnology* 18 (2000): 1018–19.

12. Whole Foods, "Genetically Engineered Food" (undated), http://www.whole foodsmarket.com/values/genetically-engineered.php (accessed December 16, 2009).

13. William Neuman, "'Non-GMO' Seal Identifies Foods Mostly Biotech-Free," *New York Times,* August 28, 2009; "Alarmed that genetically engineered crops may be finding their way into organic and natural foods an industry group has begun a campaign to test products and label [them] . . . The organic and natural foods industry is like 'a dirty room' in need of cleaning").

14. Hansen, "Does Autonomy Count?"

15. U.S. Food and Drug Administration, *Draft Guidance on Voluntary Labeling Indicating Whether Foods Have or Have Not Been Developed Using Bioengineering,* 2001, http://www.fda.gov/Food/GuidanceComplianceRegulatoryInformation/Guidance Documents/FoodLabelingNutrition/ucm059098.htm (accessed December 16, 2009).

16. *Organic and Non-GMO Report,* "Non-GMO Labels Found on Many Foods," September 2008.

17. http://www.nongmoproject.org (accessed December 16, 2009).

18. See, for example, Canadian General Standards Board, *Voluntary Labelling and Advertising of Foods that Are and Are Not Products of Genetic Engineering,* 2004, http://www.tpsgc-pwgsc.gc.ca/cgsb/on_the_net/032_0315/standard-e.html (accessed September 15, 2009).

19. K. A. Goldman, "Labeling of Genetically Modified Foods: Legal and Scientific Issues," *Georgetown International Environmental Law Review* 12 (2000): 717–60.

20. See G. P. Sampson, *The WTO and Sustainable Development* (Tokyo: United Nations University Press, 2005; emphasis added).

Conclusion

1. M. Mansour and S. Key, "From Farm to Fork: The Impact on Global Commerce of the New European Union Biotechnology Regulatory Scheme," *International Lawyer* 38 (2004): 55–70.

2. Ibid.

3. G. Conko, "Eat, Drink, and Be Merry: Why Mandatory Biotech Food Labeling Is Unnecessary," Cascade Policy Institute, October 2002.

Appendix A: Animal Cloning

1. For example, scientists have cloned cats that "glow in the dark." Australian Broadcasting Corporation, "Scientists Clone Glow-in-the-Dark Cats," December 13, 2007, http://www.abc.net.au/science/articles/2007/12/13/2118028.htm?site=science&topic=latest (accessed September 15, 2009.

2. R. Weiss, "FDA Is Set to Approve Milk, Meat from Clones," *Washington Post,* October 17, 2006, A1.

3. U.S. Food and Drug Administration, *Animal Cloning: A Risk Assessment,* 2008, http://www.fda.gov/cvm/cloneriskassessment_final.htm (accessed September 15, 2009).

4. National Research Council, *Animal Biotechnology: Science Based Concerns* (Washington, D.C.: National Academy Press, 2002).

5. European Food Safety Authority, "EFSA Adopts Final Scientific Opinion on Animal Cloning," press release, July 24, 2008, http://www.efsa.europa.eu/EFSA/efsa_locale-1178620753812_1211902019762.htm (accessed September 15, 2009).

6. Consumers Union, "Consumers Union Calls on Congress to Require Tracking and Labeling of Clones for Milk and Meat," press release, January 17, 2008, http://www.consumersunion.org/campaigns//notinmyfood/005685indiv.html (accessed September 15, 2009). The poll conducted by Consumers Union, a strong proponent of mandatory labeling for products from cloned animals, found that 89 percent want such labels and that 69 percent were concerned about eating milk or meat from cloned animals.

7. See U.S. Food and Drug Administration, Center for Veterinary Medicine, "CVM and Animal Cloning," January 15, 2008, http://www.fda.gov/cvm/cloning.htm (accessed September 15, 2009).

8. U.S. Senate, *Cloned Food Labeling Act,* S.414, 110th Cong., 1st sess., 2007.

9. See Doug Mosebar, "Legislative Scorecard Underscores the Importance of Farm Team," California Farm Bureau, 2007, http://www.cfbf.com/pdf/Scorecard2007.pdf (accessed September 15, 2009).

10. See R. Weiss, "Labels Weighed for Food From Clones," *Washington Post,* January 20, 2008, A9.

11. A. Madrigal, "Cloning Companies Promise to Track Their Animals," *Wired Science,* December 20, 2007, http://blog.wired.com/wiredscience/2007/12/cloning-compani.html (accessed September 15, 2009).

About the Authors

Gary E. Marchant is the Lincoln Professor of Emerging Technologies, Law, and Ethics at the Sandra Day O'Connor College of Law at Arizona State University in Tempe, Arizona. He is also a professor in the School of Life Sciences at ASU and the executive director of ASU's Center for Law, Science & Innovation, and he directs the nation's first LLM (Master of Laws) program in genomics and biotechnology law. Professor Marchant has a PhD in genetics from the University of British Columbia, a Master of Public Policy degree from the Kennedy School of Government, and a law degree from Harvard Law School. Prior to joining the ASU faculty in 1999, he was a partner in the Washington, D.C., office of the law firm Kirkland and Ellis. Professor Marchant teaches and researches in the subject areas of environmental law, risk assessment and risk management, genetics and the law, biotechnology law, nanotechnology law, and law, science, and technology.

Guy A. Cardineau is the Associated Students of Arizona State University (ASASU) Centennial Professor and a research professor emeritus in the Biodesign Institute, the School of Life Sciences, and the Sandra Day O'Connor College of Law at Arizona State University, where he is also a faculty fellow in the Center for Law, Science & Innovation, and is professor and director, Centro de Agrobiotecnología, Departamento de Biotecnología e Ingeniería de Alimentos, Tecnológico de Monterrey. He holds a PhD in molecular and cellular biology. Before moving to ASU in 2003, Dr. Cardineau spent nearly twenty years in industrial agricultural biotechnology. His efforts, collectively with members of his research team, have resulted in several products in the marketplace and in development, including Herculex Insect Resistant Corn, Widestrike Cotton, and the first plant-made pharmaceutical approved and licensed by a regulatory authority anywhere in the world, a Newcastle Disease Virus subunit vaccine produced in tobacco cell culture. He currently serves as an advisor or consultant to the startup biotechnology companies ERAbiotech, Algal Technologies, and Sonora Transplants, is a member of the Flinn Foundation BioAg Research/ Technology Platform Committee, and serves on the U.S. Department of Agriculture Advisory Committee on Biotechnology and 21st Century Agriculture (AC21). He is an inventor of twenty-five issued and fourteen published pending U.S. patent applications in the plant sciences, with over sixty patents worldwide.

Thomas P. Redick is the principal attorney in the Global Environmental Ethics Counsel law firm in St. Louis, Missouri, representing clients in the high-technology and agricultural biotechnology industry sectors. A 1985 graduate of the University of Michigan Law School, he handles legal issues relating to global regulatory approval, liability avoidance, and compliance with industry standards addressing socioeconomic and environmental impacts of multinational operations. His practice emphasizes transportation issues for high-technology recycling, hazardous waste handling, and agricultural biotechnology. Since 1998, he has represented the American Soybean Association, U.S. Soybean Export Council, and United Soybean Board in negotiations with biotech seed companies relating to domestic identity preservation and liability prevention, as well as negotiations of traceability and liability under the Cartagena Protocol on Biosafety.